Aromatherapy from Provence

D0949165

Nelly Grosjean

Aromatherapy from Provence

Translated from the French
by Margaret G. Gray

INDEX COMPILED BY
LYN GREENWOOD

SAFFRON WALDEN
THE C.W. DANIEL COMPANY LIMITED

First published in France in 1992 by Edition Vie Arôme
under the title "aromatherapy: essential oils for your health"

This edited and revised English-language edition
first published in Great Britain in 1993
by the C.W. Daniel Company Ltd
1 Church Path, Saffron Walden
Essex, CB10 1JP, England

ISBN O 85207 266 X

Design and Typesetting by Yew Design
Produced in association with Book Production Consultants plc, Cambridge
Printed in England by St Edmundsbury Press, Bury St Edmunds, Suffolk

Also by Nelly Grosjean

(all in French)

Aromathérapie, soigner grâce aux essences de plantes.
Edition Chiron

Aromathérapie 2, des huiles essentielles pour votre santé.
Edition Vie Arôme.

Aromathérapie esthétique, des huiles essentielles beauté-santé.
Edition Vie Arôme.

Aromathérapie, des huiles essentielles dans votre assiette,
l'alimentation gagneur.
Edition Vie Arôme.

Aromathérapie vétérinaire.
Edition la Chevêche.

100 remèdes d'urgences. In preparation.
Edition la Chevêche.

La cuisine aromatique en provence
In preparation.

L'aromatherapie Santé et Bien Etre par les huiles essentielles
Edition Albin Michel

Contents

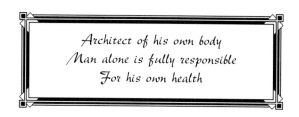

Architect of his own body
Man alone is fully responsible
For his own health

HEALTH
IS A
BALANCE

between

what is taken in

air (inspiration)

water

food

thought (positive)

what is given out

CO2 (expiration)

urine

stools

relaxation (negative)

Foreword

The advocates of natural health have been waiting for a long time for a synthesis of this science which is a major art deriving from orthodox naturopathy; aromatherapy.

Nelly Grosjean is one of the major contemporary specialists in aromatherapy*. Her reputation and expertise have become known across the Atlantic. This is an essential tool for anyone wanting a serious but practical reference book with guidelines to the application of this wonderful natural health technique.

Today there are many para-naturopathic and eclectic methods seeking entry into the field of natural health, but they lack a clear, well-formulated approach. This could only come from an orthodox and highly respected naturopath who was trained in the best schools. Nelly Grosjean has produced an accurate and honest book, which takes the art of aromatherapy out of the realm of improvisation and uncertainty. This is a significant work, a book not to be ignored.

I hope that this dynamic, enthusiastic and competent woman will play an important role in the evolution of orthodox naturopathy, which is the only global and fundamental medicine.

On behalf of my North American, European and international colleagues, I congratulate Nelly Grosjean on the publication of this work, which marks an important date in the evolution of her profession and the health of mankind.

Dr Jean-Marc BRUNET N.D., D.Sc., PhD.
Rector, Susan B Anthony University (U.S.A.)

* Nelly Grosjean, N.D., Doctor of Naturopath, Susan B Antony University, Missouri, U.S.A.

Definitions

AROMATHERAPY IS ETYMOLOGICALLY THE TREATMENT OF
AILMENTS (THERAPY) WITH AROMAS (ESSENCES OR
ESSENTIAL OILS OF AROMATIC PLANTS).

AROMATHERAPY IS ONE OF THE TECHNIQUES OF HOLISTIC,
ALTERNATIVE OR NATURAL MEDICINE.

AROMATHERAPY CAN BE AS MUCH PREVENTATIVE
AS CURATIVE.

AROMATHERAPY ABOVE ALL, 'HEALS', REALIGNS AND
RE-BALANCES THE WHOLE BODY.

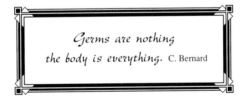

*Germs are nothing
the body is everything.* C. Bernard

The Ten Golden Rules for Well-Being

> *Respect is the royal road to self-fulfilment,*
> *Which is attainable only through self-knowledge*

I have always been drawn to these 'golden rules for well-being', and it seems reasonable to restate them at the start of this book. They never change, and it is only by practicing them that we can experience the beneficial effects they have upon our physical, mental and spiritual health.

Presented simply, clearly and precisely as a set of golden rules, here are aromatherapy's precepts and essential principles for healthy living.

They have to be followed daily to nurture our health and also to avoid disease and increase our essential vitality, energy and 'joie de vivre'.

These golden rules are valid for children and adults, to the well or the sick, and for men and women alike. Their purpose is to bring healthy, sometimes new habits into the home.

The Ten Golden Rules for Health and Beauty

by Nelly Grosjean

1. Nourishment
2. Breathing
3. Physical Exercise
4. Relaxation
5. Sleep
6. Water Intake
7. Sunshine
8. Sexual and Emotional Balance
9. Aromatherapy
10. Positive Thinking

- Healthy, well-balanced eating
  (Raw food, one main meal, quiet mind)
  Good elimination: drink to evacuate
  Drop the work 'diet' from your vocabulary
- Breathe deeply for three minutes night and morning and as often as possible during the day
- A little physical exercise every day, or take part in a sport of your choosing several times a week. Approach this gradually with a period of rest and recuperation to follow
- 5 to 10 minutes of relaxation will recharge your batteries
- Hours of sleep before midnight have double the value
- A cool shower every morning
- A warm shower or bath every evening
- Have 'air bath' and 'sun baths' as often as possible
- Give some thought every day to creating harmony with your partner
- Aromatise the air you breathe with an aroma diffuser and have aromatic frictions every morning and evening
- Smile to yourself every single morning. Do at least one positive thing and think at least one positive thought every day

Hygiene for a Healthy Life

All living species stand in direct relationship to the movements of the universe, through their structures, their shapes and their tissues.

Nutrition

1. EAT HEALTHY FOOD
whenever possible free of additives and chemicals
– large quantities of fresh vegetables, raw rather than cooked; large quantities of vegetable juice
– raw fresh fruit, between meals always.
Without eating beforehand, 10am and 4pm are the ideal times to take raw fruit.
Cooked fruit (stewed or even baked apples without sugar) make excellent desserts
– one protein dish per meal: egg, fish, poultry, meat, milk-based dish or cereal
– good quality seasonings: cold-pressed virgin oils, sea salt, lemon or cider vinegar, natural yoghurts, cream cheeses.
2. TAKE TIME OVER A MEAL, if possible in peaceful surrounds.
3. REMEMBER TO CHEW and salivate.
4. WATCH FOR GOOD ELIMINATION.
5. DRINK AT LEAST 1½ LITRES OF WATER PER DAY between meals, either water or a warm or cold infusion, or water with hydrosols.*

Diet: Errors and foods to avoid

a) Number one enemy: sugar and its derivatives: sweets, chocolate, cakes, syrups and ice-cream. The sugar from our daily intake of fruit is enough for our needs.
b) Bread, rice, pasta, white flour: wholly devitalised food. You could make wallpaper glue with the starch in them. Imagine their effect upon your body!
c) Commercially produced jams, cold meats, pre-cooked meals: heavy to digest; all too often prepared in a sauce containing chemical additives!
d) Wines, spirits, tea and coffee are stimulants which become addictive. The habit should be broken!
e) Avoid too much meat: twice a day is too much.
f) Avoid too much cheese. It causes rheumatism!

*see page 13

History of Aromatherapy

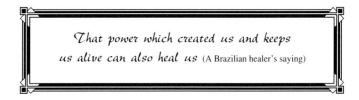

> *That power which created us and keeps*
> *us alive can also heal us* (A Brazilian healer's saying)

In 1984 researchers working in different parts of the world made the following discoveries:
– DNA synthesis
– the life atom and the death atom
– that the cell is sensitive to electromagnetic waves
– many synthetic drugs, which can be made from one of the scientifically insolated, active elements of a plant
– 'a posteriori' discovery of the secondary reactions of the human body to synthetic drugs. Some of them found to be dangerous 30 years after being intensively used (DDT, Thalidomide)
– the active properties manifested by the various elements which make up a plant; the active properties of isolated elements are not the same as those of the whole of the plant from which they are extracted.

Computer science opens up enormous new possibilities in medical science, chemistry, biology and pharmacology. Since the beginning of time plants have been in general use for medical treatment. The World Health Organization (WHO) has declared that numerous investigations should be made into the knowledge of healers, herbalists and sorcerers all over the world so that scientific tests can be carried out to corroborate their empirical knowledge (1983 WHO statement).

Let's find out about the history of plants and essential oils by taking a trip through time and through different civilisations and parts of the world.

In India

The first medical documents, Tsacharaka-Samhida, dates back to 1,000 years BC.

The Atharweda, a major book which is still consulted, talks of the respiratory energies of plants. Medical treatments were brought together in this book after the Aryan invasions.

In China

Tradition tells us that the God Emperor Shgen Nung, who rules China 2838 to 2698 BC gave men botanical science.

Confucius (c. 455–479 BC), the most famous of the Chinese philosophers, extolled the "theory of vital energy and breathing", wrote "treatise of the bedroom" about sexual harmony and hygiene, and formulated laws of hygiene, the salutary use of baths, showers and massage, telling us that "coitus" means "battle with flowers".

Tsao-Tchouan (c. 540 BC) and the Han Dynasty refer back to medicine "beyond the Century of Iron to the Saints and Sages of the Golden Age".

During the Mandarin era "a great physician does not treat what is already sick, he treats that which is not yet sick". (Old Chinese proverb).

In Egypt

Marjoram is attributed to Osiris, armoise to Isis, marrube to Horus and chamomile to the sun.

The medical principles of the Pharaohs' Egypt are brought together in the 'Ebers' papyri found in Thebes in 1873. At any point in time men were seeking 'the miracle cure'. Polydamno found the "magical sap, pain and anger-soothing, which overcomes all ills." Papyri dating back to 2800 BC bear witness that:

"oregano, cinnamon, juniper and mint were used in ointments and creams prepared by pressing out the essence of herbs or by macerating them in fatty oils".

"In temples, precious ointments and fragrant essences". Fragrant essences were used to embalm high-ranking Egyptians.

Preparation of essences, oils and flowers, 2800 BC, the era when plant oils were first expressed in Egypt.

In Greece

Theophrastes wrote 'The Treatises of Odours'. Is this a new departure or a continuation of the development of aromatherapy throughout the ages?

Chiron, sage and centaur cured Pheonix of his blindness with medicinal herbs, one of which was centaurea. At the same time Aesculapius, the Greek god of medicine, was healing with "words, medicinal herbs and a blade", so says Pindar. Hence Asclepiades, or physician priests. In terms of the history of medicine the methods were primitive, limited to a few phytotherapeutic treatments, elementary physiology and some surgery.

Was Heraclios the first hygienist? He advocated warm hydrotherapy and medicinal herbs. And Melampsos – king of Pylos and also a physician – was already practising metallotherapy, curing Iphides of his impotence with iron oxide.

Aesculapius, as a physician and son of Apollo, and himself the god of medicine, could raise the dead. Maybe his statues as the son of god has given him Jesus Christs's powers.

Panaceos was a renowned healer who gave her name to the word panacea, a universal remedy. Panaceos, daughter of Aesculapius and granddaughter of Apollo, was also a Greek divinity.

Hippocrates (5th Century BC) is the father of medicine as we all know it. His famous oath is still taken by doctors at the start of their careers.

Aristotle and Theophrastes were his students. Dioscordies (1st century BC) had a very great influence on botanists of the Renaissance period.

Pliny and Gallienus succeeded Dioscorides and extended the range of his work.

In Greece: 'Treatise of Odours' by Theophrastes.

In Persia

Avicenna (980 AD) in his own 'Canon of Medicine' relates that "while studying medicinal plants he discovered how to prepare the volatile essences of flowers and plants by the process of distillation". His 'Canon of Medicine' was at the time the principal reference work for both Muslims and Europeans.

In Persia Avicenna was the inventor of distillation.

In Rome

Aromatic oils were used in youth elixirs and Heracles' sacred plant was the poplar.

In the Middle Ages

Physicians were still priests. Pope Innocent III issued a Papal decree by which no ecclesiastic was allowed to practise medicine for money or to shed any blood at all. Physician monks thus began cultivating herbal gardens, and became apothecaries (they left their orders) or healers who sold their potions in towns and villages. Physician priests who remain within the Church's fold passed on their medical duties to barbers, as the physician diagnosed without touching the patient, through his urine and his horoscope, and sent his instructions to an apothecary. The treatment of the sick took account of the writings of Hippocrates, involving the four constitutions: sanguine, phlegmatic, bilious, melancholic; and the four moods: blood:air, phlegm:water, bile:fire, and atrabilious:earth. In China it was based on Yin and Yang and the theory of the five elements.

The 16th century sees the doctrine of similars (law or similitude) and the examination of the cause of the illness to find a treatment: one of the bases of homoeopathy.

The majority of drugs were vegetable-based and alchemy allowed great progress in chemistry and metallurgy. The search of the elixir of eternal life has always given scholars occasion to surpass themselves.

The external and internal use of aromatic herbal oils figures in some texts from the 16th century and before, corresponding to what we know today of aromatherapy.

Essential Oils were seen in those days as the pure spirit of a plant, thus influencing mind and emotions as well as the physical body. Dew from herbs, special methods of breathing and exercising were used, and music was considered particularly beneficial, alto, tenor, bass and soprano being placed in parallel with the four moods.

Preventative medicine was supremely important, especially where diet was concerned, in accordance with Hippocrates' good old principle: "Let food be your medicine".

Aromatic essential oils
for external or internal use were in the Middle Ages
"the pure spirit of a plant".

Little by little medicine and botany progressed, as the power of the Church over physicians declined.

Then Came the 20th Century

The awakening of modern medicine, the work of P. and M. Curie, C. Bernard, and Pasteur with his astonishing assertion: "Germs are nothing, the body is all" point out the new road to be followed: the study and knowledge of the body present as much interest if not more than the study of germs... But we have to go very far back in time to discover the real origins of today's naturopathic medicine, the treatment of the whole person. In fact we have to go back to the Sumerian.

50 Centuries Ago

Surgeons, herbalists, naturopaths and priests were learned physicians who treated "the spirit to heal the body", and discovered that 'darkness' (the word 'illness' did not exist) was a 'curative crisis' in preparation for the birth of the spirit. (Document found on the site of the ruined Sumerian city of Nippur.)

Sumerian sacred medicine, according to Marguerite Enderlin, an eminent French sumerologist, contains astonishing elements which tend to prove that naturopaths and practitioners of 'soft' medicine had famous precursors: scholars who worked in astrology, phytotherapy, anatomy, pharmacopoeia, diagnosis and prognosis, the practice of hepatoscopy, secret sciences which gave them the ability to interpret dreams, colours and oil stains on water.

The Sumerian physician-priest was a miracle worker, who knew how to escort his patient down to hell and back. The secret, initiatory teaching passed on to each Sumerian physician has not yet been deciphered from tablets and perhaps it will remain thus forever unbroken.

Following a spiritual preparation based on meditation and prayer the Sumerian physician started with a clinical examination of the patient; his stature, gait, aggression, mental disorders, temperature, eye quality, retina, urine, elasticity of muscles, small of the back; then observation and deduction from the state of organs and analysis of internal pains; lastly examination of head and bones.

The Sumerian physician knew the importance of accentuating or ameliorating rhythms and administered his medication at set times, at dawn, twilight or at night, according to each individual case.

Other stone tablets mention the critical periods of any given disease and its cyclic or successive phases and predict the number of days until either a fatal issue or fully recovery. On some tablet dating back over 4,000 years, diagnoses and medical prescriptions can also be found.

Frictions and the inhalation of essences
were practiced over 4,000 years ago!

Aromatherapy, oligosols and lithotherapy (crushed stones) were used every day in Sumer in remotest antiquity: treatments in which all techniques were utilised. Any physicians were "specialists in all matters", practicing medicine for the whole person, physical, spiritual and holistic...

On this level the new orthodox naturopathic doctors, be they energists, acupuncturists or hypnotists, link up with Sumerian sacred medicine. Only a few years ago we did not know that frictions with essential oils were in everyday use in those days to maintain good health, re-establish the proper circulation of the 'breath of life' = a vital energy and stimulate 're-vitalisation' = healing. The role of the Sumerian physician was to allow his patient to recover 'the light of glory' and the 'the heart's secret' = good health! Man, as he evolved between his phases of 'light' = good health and 'dark' = disease, was allowed to get closer to immortality. This state of equilibrium is close to Hindu and Tibetan writings on the external evolution of Being through moral and physical trails.

The Sumerian physician, the Tibetan lama and the Muslim priest were entrusted with his high and glorious task: to help man in his spiritual progress by maintaining his physical condition and his psyche.

Let us hope the doctors do not forget the full and complete range of their task; only then shall we benefit from whole medicine, a medicine for man in his full spiritual and physical being, and not a medicine of symptoms which cuts man up in slices, each specialist treating only the parts he has elected to treat... A medicine which treats the body as a whole, a medicine for the physical, psychic and spiritual bodies. Tomorrow's medicine, towards which we are progressing in great strides for the good of all.

A human medicine!
Orthodox Naturopathy!
Holistic medicine!

And finally, the oldest known relationship between man and plants: more than 60,000 years ago primitive man buried his dead covered in flowers! (Excavations in the Shanidar caves.)

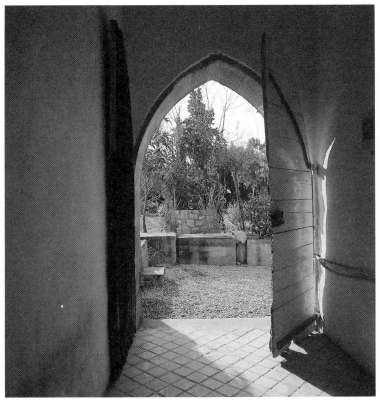

An open door on health...
La Chevêche, Graveson en Provence.

Essential Oil

Essential oil is the noble (or first) yield from the distillation of an aromatic plant. An aromatic plant is a plant which contains sufficient quantities of aromatic and odoriferous elements to be distilled.

Not all plants yield essential oils. However all plants can be distilled to produce floral water, hydrosol or hydrolat. Hydrosol or hydrolat is the complementary yield to essential oil. It is obtained by distilling the plant. It contains a minute proportion of suspended aromatic matter, in sufficient quantity to have a therapeutic effect.

Hydrosol-therapy is rather like aromatherapy's homoeopathy. Often used in drinks and healthcare products, it is perfectly suitable for children, for sensitive even delicate persons and/or those who over-react whether for physical or emotional reasons. For example:
"I don't like essential oils. They burn. They are too strong." "When I take them I belch. I feel as if my stomach is burning..." etc.

Aromatherapy and hydrosoltherapy are applied primarily in the daily diet.
How?
– in seasonings (salads, sauces, cereals)
– in drinks (hot or cold)
– in a healthy nutritious drink: the 'health drinks'
– in treatments: 'cocktails', 'toddies'...
– in daily health frictions

Hydrosol: Homoeopathy or Alchemy of an Aroma?

Hydrosol is 'our' designation for hydrolat or floral water from a distillation with spring water, from which only the first 20 litres are collected. During distillation water is heated and passes steam through the plants, carrying aromatic elements with it before it is cooled. The essential oil separates from the floral water in the still because of a density differential.

Hydrosols can be obtained from all existing plants, even the non-aromatic ones (oak, beech, fenugreek, holly, boxwood, plantain, fern), but only 'aromatic' plants will yield essential oil.

The aromatic elements suspended in water, together with the water, produce an hydrolat. As soon as these aromatic elements are in sufficient quantity to separate out from the water, they form the essential oil, or essence, which floats on the surface of the distillation water. Aromatic molecules, when there are enough to them, create aromatic essential oil.

The plant's aromatic properties come from small 'aroma sacs' in aromatic plants, which are 'exploded' in the distillation process. Steam carries them into the distillation water, from which they will be separated in the essential oil still. In the case of citrus fruit these 'aroma sacs' can also be opened mechanically (i.e. in the zest of: lemon, orange, bergamot, mandarin and grapefruit).

Synergy

Synergy means the combination of several factors, whose united action creates a single (new) effect.

The therapeutic potential of natural products is altered by synergy. Synergy creates mysterious new properties, which cannot be wholly explained by the sum of the parts.

The synergy of essential oils thus creates a 'new product' with different properties, with a therapeutic potential which may be stronger, more selective, more efficient or simply different...

$$1 + 1 = 3$$

N.B. When using the prescriptions on the following pages, i.e. when taking by mouth:

Essential oil (1 to 3 drops) can be taken in a spoonful of honey or in a glass of hot, not boiling water.

The ideal way is to put a drop of essential oil on the back of your hand and lick it off. This is an easy, practical way to take a full dose in the office or while travelling.

Rather than using many different essential oils for a specific purpose, it is always better to use just one or to have an already blended mixture made up by a specialist. Don't play the alchemist!

The Plateau Effect*

One of the things which I must emphasize most strongly is how important it is to use small doses and treatments of brief duration; and how vitally important it is to change the essential oils during a aromatherapy treatment to accord with the changes brought about in the body. When using essential oils these changes occur rapidly.

This is illustrated by the Plateau effect: the physiological response to any given medication. Prescribed doses will bring proportional results up to a given threshold, which varies according to the essential oil used. If the dose is increased or is having a cumulative effect, the results, which so far have been in proportion to the dose, will now be in inverse proportion. The response, that is the expected therapeutic effect, thus becomes negative, even opposite.

Throughout this book I warn against the 'blind' use of essential oils and against the noxious effect of heavy doses. It would therefore be wise to respect the dose recommended for a given pathological condition or for use as a preventative.

Summary

Low doses
+ treatments
+ change and adjustment of essential oil as a treatment proceeds
= expected therapeutic result
The aim is to encourage the practical and intelligent use of essential oils in the home by parents concerned about the proper use of aromatherapy and about a new and healthy way of life.

To maintain and increase
everyone's potential for health.

*Named after the person who discovered the 'Plateau' effect.

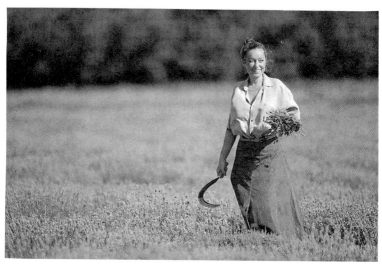

Nelly Grosjean gathering lavender with a sickle at an altitude of 1,100 metres. This biological crop is cultivated by Vie Arôme, France.

CHAPTER 1

Therapy

Different uses of Essential Oils

- – Diffusion
- – Frictions
- – Internal Uses
- – Inhalations
- – Baths
- – Other Uses

Quick reference to Everyday Essential Oils in the Home

Different Uses of Essential Oils

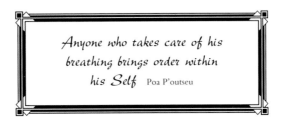

Anyone who takes care of his breathing brings order within his Self   Poa P'outseu

Diffusion in the Atmosphere

Aromatic essential oils diffused in the atmosphere by means of a diffuser permit the 'absorption through the lungs' of volatile micro-particles – the active elements – of essential oils.

Diffusing essential oils in the atmosphere is certainly the best way to benefit from them without inconvenience.

The Effect of Essential Oils in the Atmosphere

a) Eliminate any unpleasant smell

Tobacco – smoke – crowd – sanitation – cooking...

b) Revitalise – rejuvenate – re-energise the air you breathe

c) Supply negative ions

Often absent from cities and dwelling places, negative ions are best supplied by a negative ion generator. However essential oils diffused in the atmosphere do the job both adequately and agreeably.

d) Give access to the specific powers of essential oils to those who smell or breathe them in. The following oils are classified according to effect:

Respiratory

Pine, Eucalyptus, Cajuput, Niaouli, Thyme, Hyssop, Lavender.

Revitalising

Coriander, Savory, Nutmeg, Rosemary, Clove, Oregano, Rosegeranium.

Relaxing

Lavender, Marjoram, Chamomile, Orange, Petit-Grain, Neroli, Bergamot.

Exotic revitalising

Cinnamon, Sandalwood, Ylang-Ylang.

Soft and pleasant

Vervain, Rose Geranium, Rosewood, Chamomile.

The Aroma Diffuser

This is an electrical apparatus which disperses the micro-particles of essential oils into the atmosphere by vibration. By this method the essential oils are not heated and therefore retain all their properties.
Essential oils placed in the specially designed glassware nebulise in the room where the diffuser is placed.
It functions:
– at low volume: all day or all night.
– at maximum volume: 1 hour in the morning and 1 hour in the evening before going to bed.
There are various models adapted to different room sizes.

Advantages of the electrical aroma diffuser
– Essential oils are not heated.
– The air in a room is saturated with essential oil in record time – approximately 15 minutes.
– The practical side of the aroma diffuser: it can use different blends for day or night, for colder weather, or simply as a way of enhancing your home.

Operating times of the aroma diffuser
– In the home: switch on at maximum for 1 hour in the morning and 1 hour at night; or else all day or all night at minimum.
– In a conference room: switch to maximum throughout the conference.
– In a office, shop, hotel lobby, doctor's surgery, reception rooms: the apparatus can function non-stop.
– For better sleep: switch on for 1 hour in the room before going to bed.
– During the winter: switch on non-stop in all living rooms.

Incense Burners: Oil lamps

Perfume the atmosphere but do not have a significant therapeutic action. However the diffusion of essential oils by this means perfumes the atmosphere at the same time as making it pleasant.
A few drops of essential oil on lamps or in saucers
On a radiator they cleanse and perfume the atmosphere in a way that is simple, practical and cheap, especially respiratory oils in winter; or on lamps, anti-mosquito oils in summer.

Pot Pourri Diffuser

To a pretty bowl filled with dried flowers add a few drops of your essential oils (approximately 100 drops = 1 small spoon, monthly).

Summary: Breathing air charged with essential oils would be sufficient to prevent many epidemics, chills; would be conducive to relaxation and energy and would introduce cellular harmony into your body: good health factor – joie de vivre, happiness! 'Bonheur'.

For Diffusion, the Best-loved and Most Exotic Essential Oil

The essential oil of happiness, Vervain, is much loved by everyone in all circumstances.

The list of essential oils which are pleasant when diffused is to be found in the table on 'Use of the Main Essential Oils".

There are many recipes for excellent blends in the following chapters: Cajuput, Chamomile, Cedar, Coriander, Eucalyptus, Rosegeranium, Hyssop, Lavender, Marjoram, Mint, Orange, Oregano, Rosemary, Sage, Thyme, Vervain.

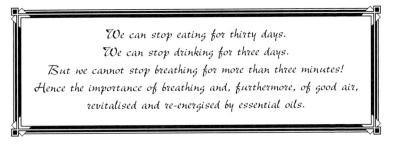

> We can stop eating for thirty days.
> We can stop drinking for three days.
> But we cannot stop breathing for more than three minutes!
> Hence the importance of breathing and, furthermore, of good air, revitalised and re-energised by essential oils.

Frictions, with Aromatic Oils*

When the Egyptians started using essential oils other than for embalming it was for frictions. They were appreciated for their fragrance as much as for their medical properties.

Why Use Essential Oil in Frictions?

We know that after essential oils have been applied to the skin they penetrate the blood and lymph within four hours.

Furthermore the exceptional ability of essential oils to select has the following advantage: essential oils in frictions on any part of the body will be inevitably attracted by the weak organ or the disturbed function.

General precaution: avoid mucous membrane and genitalia.

*See 'Frictions with Essential Oils' on page 79 & 80 to verify.

We shall first discuss the 'health frictions', which anyone can use to increase his vital potential, and which help the body to wake in the morning and relax and sleep well at night.
– Tonic frictions
– Relaxing frictions
– Digestive frictions
– Circulatory frictions
– 'Anti-pain' frictions (pain killers)
– Aphrodisiac frictions
Then the following specific frictions:
– Skin frictions
– Foot frictions
– Hair frictions

General Dosage

Body frictions	30 drops
Stomach and abdomen frictions	10 to 20 drops
Pain frictions	4 to 10 drops
Leg frictions	10 to 20 drops
Foot frictions	10 drops
Hair frictions	50 to 100 drops
Face frictions	5 to 7 drops
Chest and back frictions	20 to 30 drops

For children with very delicate skin: frictions are always mixed with an identical volume of Wheat germ, sweet almond or olive oil.

Special precautions
Never use frictions on infants (6 months or younger)

In aromatherapy we prefer to use small, regular doses...
and treatments lasting 3 to 6 weeks...
Only a few essential oils can be used by themselves or in blends without being diluted.
The other essential oils must be mixed in small quantities with at least one of the oils listed below, or mixed with wheat germ, sweet almond or olive oil, in a neutral body milk or even in essential oil of Lavender.

Natural and non-diluted

Rosewood	Cajuput	Chamomile
Caraway	Cedar	Lemon
Cypress	Eucalyptus	Juniper
Rosegeranium	Lavender	Marjoram
Niaouli	Orange	Petitgrain
Pine	Rosemary	Sandalwood
Ylang-ylang		

Mixed or diluted

Green aniseed	Basil	Bergamot
Cinnamon	Coriander	Tarragon
Ginger	Clove	Lemongrass
Mint	Nutmeg	Neroli
Oregano	Rose	Savory
Sassafras	Sage	Turpentine
Thuja	Thyme	Vervain

Special precautions: with Mint, Thyme, Oregano, Clove and Ginger –
use maximum 1:10 blends.

Finally, the mixing of essential oils will have to be done carefully as
indicated below.
Various methods exist, but in any case it is advisable:
– never to mix more than three essential oils together (unless you have
intimate knowledge of their respective synergies). (See: Synergies,
Definition, or follow the advice of your aromatherapist.)
– to adhere strictly to the specific instructions given in this book.
Example: for a respiratory problem
It is better to have a good eucalyptus friction alone than an erroneous
mixture of all essential oils labelled 'respiratory'.
The efficiency of any mixture is often superior to the use of one single oil.

When to Use Frictions

Morning, between 6am and midday	Morning tonics
Evening, between 6pm and midnight	Evening relaxation
5pm and before going to bed	Aphrodisiac
10am, 5pm and before going to bed	Circulatory
After meals	Digestive
Morning and evening	Respiratory and pain relief
Morning, 5pm and before going to bed	Circulatory
Morning and evening	Feet

How to Apply Frictions

First method:
Take a few drops of the chosen blend in your hand.
Rub your two hands together and spread on the area to be treated,
massaging/rubbing in a clockwise direction.
Second method:
Put the drops on the area to be treated and rub as above.

Where to Use Frictions

On the whole body:

Chest, neck, spine, arms, legs, soles of feet and solar plexus	Tonic, Relaxing, Aphrodisiac
Chest, neck, back and solar plexus	Respiratory
Stomach, abdomen and solar plexus	Digestive
Any painful area and solar plexus	Anti-pain
Feet, legs up to the hips	Circulatory
Feet only	Foot
Scalp	Hair
Face only	Face

The last three are more relevant to a 'cosmetic' than an 'aromatherapic' application.

For every problem frictions are more effective when – without changing the specific composition – a friction on the solar plexus is added.

Main Principles

General Dosages

INTERNAL USES

– 1 to 3 drops of essential oil or blend 2 to 5 times per day is the average dose

– except for special medical prescriptions.

– Courses of treatment of up to 3 weeks maximum with the same essential oil or blend.

Directions for use:

- In the past it was recommended that essential oils be taken on sugar. This was a bad habit since sugar, even brown, is a 'poison' to the nerve cells.
- We recommend taking essential oils in a sugar substitute, honey, which is a good vehicle for their absorption and assimilation.
- The second-best way to absorb essential oils is to take them in a large glass of warm water. They do not mix or become diluted in water.
- However, of the three prescribed drops, half to one drop will remain in the glass and not be used. The rest will be swallowed.

How to take essential oils: 7 good methods

1) Place on the back of the hand, 1 to 3 drops of essential oil and lick up, then drink a large glass of warm water or an infusion, or eat a large spoonful of honey or yoghurt to 'get rid of the taste'.

2) Take 1 to 3 drops in a spoonful of good quality honey – not heated.

3) Take 1 to 3 drops in a large glass of warm or hot water: it should not be boiling, as the volatile and subtle aromatic elements of the essential oils deteriorate in the heat.

4) Drinks containing essential oils. You will find the relevant recipes under these headings, using the following essential oils:

Anti-tobacco	Sassafras
Anti-flu	Oregano, Thyme, Eucalyptus
Pleasant drinks	Lemon, Orange, Pine
Drinks for indigestion	Oregano
Memory cocktail	Ginger, Savory
Asthma cocktail	Thyme
Aphrodisiac drinks	Ginger, Savory, Coriander

5) Pearls or capsules can also be prescribed by your aromatherapist. Capsules keep essential oils odourless and tasteless.

Intestinal capsules have both advantages and disadvantages, which your aromatherapist will assess. However there is another drawback: the protection afforded by the sense of taste is lost and it would be possible to take them in large quantities without noticing anything wrong.

For example: nothing prevents you taking ten capsules of thyme all at once – except your own good sense – but it is absolutely impossible to take ten drops of essential oil of thyme, since even one is very difficult to swallow.

6) Essential oils in a solution of alcohol can be prepared on prescription by your pharmacist.

7) Many essential oils can be used in cookery: Thyme, Rosemary, Savory, Juniper, Caraway, Cumin, Nutmeg, Aniseed, Fennel, Coriander, Sage, Ginger: in savory dishes.

Lemon, Orange, Grapefruit, Mandarin, Bergamot, Cinnamon, Ginger, Rosegeranium: in sweet dishes.

Refer to a few good recipes at the end of this book: Chapter 4, Essential Oils in the Kitchen.

Remembering that by getting close to a de-mineralised person you will be 'relieved of your mineral salts in his/her favour, it should be sufficient to touch essential oils for them to have an effect upon you.

Without carrying this empirical and esoteric, though not inaccurate theory to extremes, let us remember that taking or being in contact with essential oils in small doses several times a day is preferable to a daily dose taken once. The results depend on the size and regularity of the doses.

You will find in the glossary in this book precise instructions on essential oils and how to use them for particular illnesses. You will find tables, with dosages, frequency and length of treatments in the attached pages.

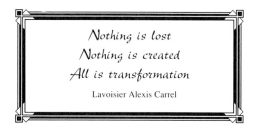

Internal Use

1) Place 1 drop of essential oil on the back of the hand and lick; the simplest and most practical method. Make sure that the oils you take internally are organic and of the highest quality; such as those from Vie Arôme.

2) For children: hydrosols (soft aromatherapy) i.e. distilled water containing suspended aromatic elements - preferable to essential oils except on the advice of an aromatherapist.

3) For infants: Never use any essential oil for internal treatment. For frictions use hydrosols of lavender, pine, eucalyptus...

Never use essential oil frictions on infants

In prescriptions the oils will always be diluted and mixed with Wheat germ oil.

– Lavender is the infants' essential oil, always diluted.

– In the case of infants you are recommended to seek the advice of your holistic physician.

Inhalations - Preparation and Use

Inhalation is one of the best and most practical ways to derive benefit from essential oils and adds to the relief given by hot steam. With an inhaler you can breathe in warm vapour saturated with essential oils.

Inhalations are used mostly for respiratory and pulmonary infections, some migraines and headaches, mainly of a nervous or digestive origin.

Warmth relaxes. The warm steam inhaled soothes coughs, clears the pulmonary tract, eases bronchial coughs, calms neuralgia. The essential oils share their own specific qualities.

Inhalations made with essential oils
- **– Soothing**   Lavender, Marjoram, Orange, Chamomile
- **– Respiratory**   Pine, Eucalyptus, Niaouli, Cajuput, Lavender, Thyme, Rosemary, Hyssop, Oregano.

Use
A few drops (3 to 10) of the chosen essential oils are placed in an inhaler, large bowl or even a saucepan of hot water.
Put your head over the inhaler or container of water, covering it with a large bath towel, so that the warm vapours are not dispersed but inhaled.

Duration of treatment
Inhalations last 3 to 7 minutes, depending upon what is bearable, and can be easily repeated 2, 3 or 4 times a day.
Flu, colds, chest infections irritating coughs, bronchitis, asthma, tuberculosis and all respiratory infections, facial neuralgia, migraine and some cephaloea - inhalations will bring relief to all of these.

Recipes
See Eucalyptus, Hyssop, Lavender, Rosemary and Thyme for dosages and specific instructions.

Aromatic Baths with Essential Oils

Cleopatra used to bathe in ass's milk. Over the centuries famous woman have taken scented baths. Early this century Abbot Kneipp used hydrotherapy in all its forms as his principal treatment: warm or cold baths, ablutions, showers of all kinds. L. Kuhne cured many diseases by strengthening the body with hip baths, frictions, foot, hand, trunk baths.

Hence through the centuries:
The significance of water and its medicinal properties
A healer after a session, without even having touched his patient, washes his hands to rid himself of 'negative or dirty vibrations' which he might have accumulated...

Water cleanses the body and the spirit
What is more relaxing than a bath or a shower after a day's work? Water not only cleanses, but it removes most of the 'invisible negative particles' which bind the spirit to the earth...

We know about the great power of water to conduct electricity. Some masseurs work with one of their hands connected to a copper wire – a power transmitter – or to a water mains. Various esoteric writings note the importance of the ability water has to discharge negative vibrations, electro-magnetic waves which act on you like electricity.

Have you ever realised that our thoughts are carried through space as '*vibrations*' or '*waves*' which may be intercepted one day, in the same way as radio or television waves are today?

Furthermore water is a generator of *negative ions* vital to the equilibrium of the air, our first 'food' for survival. Cities are overloaded with positive ions, and only waterfalls, the sea, oceans, turbulent baths, *all living waters manufacture negative ions.*

There are many examples to show the importance of water: Roman baths, hammams, Finnish saunas followed by cold baths amongst the pine forests in air charged with negative ions, Turkish baths, spa centres and, today, the craze for balneotherapy, thalassotherapy and the new Californian spa, the jacuzzi and the bubble bath...

Any 'naturopathic' or 'body-shaping' treatment is based on a good food balance, energy balance and the elimination of toxins and deficiencies.

Baths containing plant oils or, even better, aromatic baths are the sovereign remedies ('Mighty Lords') at the heart of these treatments.

Let us add to the wonderful properties of water the powers of essential oils, and then we have harmonising baths, physically and mentally balancing baths for our perturbed energies, relaxing baths, tonic baths, energising baths... baths for life!

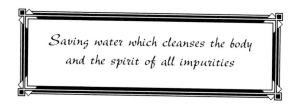

Saving water which cleanses the body and the spirit of all impurities

Other Uses

– Vaginal douches and enemas
– Hair care
– Veterinary usage

Reflexotherapy

Essential oils have been used on acupuncture points, aural and digital, for some years. Research in these areas is still being carried out.

Firstly, specific essential oils on a strategic point increase the positive effects of relaxotherapy.

Essential oils 'create' new energy.

Reflexotherapy 'balances' the energies.

Aromatherapy and reflexotherapy both belong to: 'soft' medicine, the medicine of energies, tomorrow's medicine.

Veterinary Aromatherapy

Our good friends, cats, dogs, horses, ducks, geese... can also benefit from the effects of aromatic essential oils. Many veterinary surgeons are nowadays practising aromatherapy. For cats and dogs an aroma diffuser with respiratory essential oils resolves respiratory problems. Diffusers can also be installed in stables, or by duck or goose ponds...

For dogs frictions with essential oils with give good results. Did you know that osteopathy is also being practised on animals? To deodorise a flat where cats live use an aroma diffuser with exotic vervain, mint tonic or frestonic.

Immediate results!

For dogs, to ensure a good coat, one tablespoon of yeast with all their meals, a course of chloride of magnesium three to four times a year (20g per litre of water, ½ glass twice a day), and frictions with natural essential oil of turpentine.

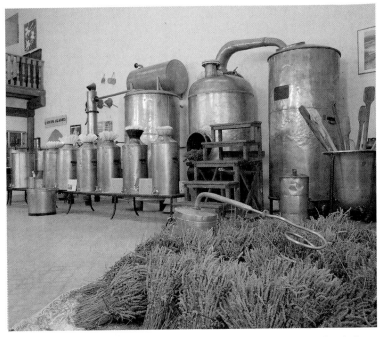

Reconstruction of a 19th Cent. distillation factory at the Musée des Arômes et du parfum, Graveson en Provence.

Quick Reference to Everyday Oils in the Home

The information given in the following pages is in summary form only. You are recommended to follow the guidance given in greater detail in other parts of this book.

The blends named below are referred to frequently in the following pages. They are manufactured by Vie Arôme. For full details see p.80–81

APH friction –	APHRODISIAC
CEL friction –	CELLULITE
DIG friction –	DIGESTIVE
HAR friction –	HARMONY
MIN friction –	SLIMMING
NER friction –	NERVOUS SYSTEM
RES friction –	RESPIRATORY
RHU friction –	RHEUMATIC
VIT friction –	VITALITY
106 friction –	For HAIR
107 friction –	For FACE
108 friction –	For CIRCULATION

Essential oils:
Chamomile, Caraway, Cinnamon, Coriander, Cypress, Eucalyptus, Juniper, Lavender, Lemon, Marjoram, Mint, Nutmeg, Orange plus Neroli, Origano, Pine, Rose/Rosewood, Sage, Sassafras, Vervain.

Caraway – Carum carvi
FOR FLATULENCE

– Intestinal oxygeniser, the best of all digestives.
Flatulence, distention, and dyspepsia.

Dosage
Internal use: 1–2 drops 3 times a day: After meals on hand, in water or honey, or licked from the hand.
External use: 5–10 drops as frictions on stomach and abdomen after meals.
Treatment: 3 times a day for 3 weeks.
Prevention: 1 treatment 2–4 times a year.

Synergies – Recipes
Internal and external use
1 drop caraway + 1 nutmeg drunk 3 times a day.
– DIGESTIVE COMPOSITION (DIG friction) or:
45ml Caraway + 30 Nutmeg + 20 Coriander + 5 Cumin: a few drops as frictions after meals.
– CULINARY AROMATHERAPY
Caraway, Cumin, Coriander, Nutmeg, Juniper, Thyme, Tarragon, Rosemary.
1–2 drops in cooked dishes to enhance flavours (stews, couscous).
Essential oil in cooking can help digest heavy meals.
– DIGESTIVE SYRUP
20 drops of Caraway + 5 Cumin + 5 Geranium + 10 Coriander + 2 Nutmeg + 1 Lavender in ½ litre alcohol (80°C) + 1½ litres sugar syrup in a warm mix (prepare syrup with 370gms) sugar for ½ litre distilled water, heat until transparent). Keep 15 to 30 days before using.

Essential oil of Caraway is the 'miracle' cure for flatulence

Chamomile – *Anthemis nobilis* or *Matricaria chamomile*

FOR SINUSITIS

– Antispasmodic
– Sinusitis, migraine, vertigo, dysmenorrhoea, irritability, allergies.

Dosage
Internal use: 1 drop 3 times a day in water or honey.
External use: frictions 10–15 drops, on temples, forehead, nape of neck, solar plexus and spine twice a day.
Treatment: during biological upset a few days internal and external use.
Prevention: diffusion in atmosphere.

Synergies – recipes
– SINUSITIS
Equal parts of Chamomile + Lavender. 3 applications a day.
– MIGRAINE, CEPHAELOEA, VERTIGO
(HAR* friction) or: 5 drops Chamomile + 5 Marjoram + 5 Mint,
2 massages per day on temples to create harmony.
– SOOTHING BATH
5 drops Chamomile + 5 Lavender in 2 tablespoons powdered milk or green seaweed.
– DIFFUSION IN ATMOSPHERE
• For allergies
• To stimulate 'harmony and creativity'
Equal parts of Chamomile + Rosewood + Cedar. To breathe all night or 2/3 hours daily.
• Harmony is the ideal composition for aroma diffusers and for yoga, meditation, creativity: it balances physical, mental and spiritual energies.
In diffusion: HARMONY
In friction: HAR Friction
– MASSAGE OIL FOR CHILDREN: 60ml Wheat Germ oil + 10 drops essential oil of Chamomile brings relaxation to delicate and 'allergic' children.

Essential oil of Chamomile is seldom used alone.

*See page 81.

Cinnamon – *Cinnamomum zeylanicum*
FOR DIARRHOEA

– **Strong antiseptic, stimulating, aphrodisiac, antispasmodic.**
Diarrhoea, colitis, impotence and frigidity.

Dosage
Internal use: 1 drop 3 times a day on hand, in water or honey.
External use: frictions and baths, always diluted in essential oil of
Lavender or Wheat germ oil.
Treatment: 3–4 times a day during crisis.
Prevention: Once a day for 3 weeks.

Synergies – Recipes
– APHRODISIAC FRICTION (APH* friction) or:
5ml Cinnamon + 10 Coriander + 15 Rosemary + 5 Clove + 5 Ginger +
15 Marjoram twice a day on solar plexus, nape of neck, spine and sole of
foot.
– APHRODISIAC MASSAGE OIL
7ml Cinnamon + 15 Rosewood + 2 Sandalwood or Ylang-ylang in 100ml
Wheat germ oil.
– DIFFUSION IN ATMOSPHERE TO 'EXOTICISE' AIR
10ml Cinnamon + 30 Cedar + 60 Lavender.
– PERFUME
– 100ml alcohol (70°C) + 10 Cinnamon + 1 Clary Sage.
– ANTI-FLU TODDY
1 drop Cinnamon + 1 Oregano + 1 Thyme + 1 Clove + 1 Geranium +
1 Ginger (optional) in a spoonful of honey + very hot water + juice of
lemon.
Taste. You can drink this 2–3 times a day with no difficulty.
– APHRODISIAC COCKTAIL AND WONDERFUL INTELLECTUAL
STIMULANT
1 drop Cinnamon (Ceylon) + 1 Savory + 1 Clove + Rosemary +
1 Geranium in a large glass of warm water, serve with ice cubes as a long
drink. A dash of mint cordial can complete this cocktail or 1 teaspoonful of
hydrosol of mint.

NOTE: 1 drop of Cinnamon every two hours stops diarrhoea.
NOTE 2: Never use Cinnamon undiluted in bath or friction – it would
set you on fire! Cinnamon burns the skin.

*See page 80.

Coriander - Coriandrum sativum
FOR STIMULATION

– **Tonic aphrodisiac, digestive**.
– All types of fatigue, dyspepsia.

Dosage
Internal use: 1 drop 3 times a day on hand, in water or honey.
External use: frictions and diffusion in atmosphere.
Treatment: Internal and external use for 3 weeks.
Prevention: 1 course of treatment once or twice a year.

Synergies – recipes
– DIGESTIVE FRICTION
See Caraway or DIG friction
– APHRODISIAC TONIC FRICTION
(APH* friction) or: 10ml coriander + 5 Cinnamon + 15 Rosemary +
5 Clove + Ginger + 15 Marjoram: a few drops in frictions twice a day on
nape of neck, solar plexus, spine and sole of feet.
– COMPOSITIONS FOR AROMA DIFFUSER
• Invigorating: Coriander + Rosemary + Juniper + Pine + Vervain +
Eucalyptus. Proportions to your liking.
• Aphrodisiac: Coriander + Ylang-ylang + Clove + Juniper + Cedar +
Nutmeg.
Proportions to your liking.
– BATHS
• Stimulating: 2 drops Coriander + 2 Juniper + 2 Rosemary in a tablespoon
of sea water or white seaweed powder.
• Aphrodisiac: 2 drops Coriander + 3 Rosewood + 1 Cinnamon in 2
tablespoons of sea water or white seaweed powder (or in milk).
– PERFUMES
Essential oil of Coriander is used in small quantities in men's perfumes.
• Coriander + Ylang-ylang + Clove
• Coriander + Mint + Oregano

NOTE: Essential oil of Coriander is a sexual and intellectual stimulant.

*See page 80.

Cypress – *Cupressus sempervirens*
FOR CIRCULATION

– Alleviates menopausal circulation (venous)
– heavy legs, haemorrhoids, varicose veins, circulatory problems, hot feet.

Dosage
Internal use: 1 drop 3 times a day on hand, in water or honey. Abstain in evening.
External use: frictions morning and at 5pm on legs and feet.
Treatment: Internal and external use for 3 weeks.
Prevention: 1 course of treatment 3 or 4 times a year.

Synergies – recipes
– MENOPAUSAL CIRCULATION AND WEAK ARTERIES AND VEINS (problems for males and females)
Internal use: 1 drop Cypress + 2 drops Lemon 3 times a day, early in the morning, 10am and 2pm + friction in the morning and in the evening with 108* and CEL* friction. Add hydrosol of Sage in your daily drinking water.
– COMPOSITION FOR 'HOT FEET'
(108* friction) or: 10ml Cypress + 15ml Sage as friction morning and evening. Prevents perspiration. Take 2 drops Lemon 3 times a day.
– COMPOSITION FOR HEAVY LEGS
10ml Cypress + 15ml Sage + 1ml Mint 10am and 5pm + friction on legs and soles of feet.
– BED WETTING
1 drop Cypress 10am and 5pm + friction on the solar plexus.
– CELLULITE
CEL* friction + 108* friction together morning and evening on feet, legs and buttocks.
+ internal use: 1 drop CEL* 3 times a day for 1 week. Alternate with 1 drop 108* 3 times a day for 6 weeks.

My advice: A course of essential oil of Cypress once or twice a year is strongly recommended for anyone with a bilious temperament as a precaution against circulatory problems. Also take a course of hydrosol of Sage!

*See page 81.

Eucalyptus – Eucalyptus globulus
FOR RESPIRATION

– No. 1 pulmonary antiseptic
– Prevents colds, flu, angina, chills, soothes cough and bronchitis.
Dosage
Internal use: 1 to 3 drops 3 times a day on hand, in water or honey.
External use: friction with 10 to 20 drops, on chest or back twice a day or RES* friction.
Treatment: Internal and external during crisis.
Prevention: for 3 weeks before winter.

Synergies – recipes
– INHALATION
2 drops Eucalyptus + 2 Pine + 1 Thyme + 5 Lavender.
3 to 7 minutes inhalation 2 – 3 times daily.
– BATHS
5 drops Eucalyptus + 5 Lavender, in 2 tablespoons of green seaweed, powdered milk or sea water (or milk).
– SPECIFIC SYNERGIES FOR INTERNAL USE TREATMENTS AND FRICTIONS
• Tracheitis   Eucalyptus + Pine
• Sinusitis   Eucalyptus + Lavender + Chamomile
• Asthma   Eucalyptus + Hyssop
• Bronchitis   Eucalyptus + Niaouli + Cajuput
• Colds   RES* friction (all respiratory problems)

Diffusion in the atmosphere
15ml Pine, 5ml Thyme, 20ml Eucalyptus, 20ml Lavender together.

My advice: As soon as you feel a chill coming on, switch on your aroma diffuser, put yourself on a diet for 1 day, take a laxative infusion, 1 or 2 inhalations + 2 frictions + 'Anti flu' toddies (see: Cinnamon) and rest in a warm room.
The next day: it's all over!

NOTE: Essential oil of Eucalyptus is a basic requirement for your natural home pharmacy.

*See page 80.

Juniper – *Juniperus communis*
FOR RHEUMATIC PROBLEMS

– **Anti-rheumatic and diuretic.**

– All rheumatic problems, water retention and slimming.

Dosage

Internal use: 1 to 2 drops 3 times a day on hand, in water or honey.

External use: frictions twice daily. Bath once daily.

Treatment: Internal and external use for 3 weeks.

Prevention and maintenance: 1 course of treatment spring and autumn.

Synergies – recipes

– SLIMMING

Internal use: 1 drop Juniper + Geranium + 1 drop Lemon twice a day on hand, in water or honey (see: Lemon).

– PAIN RELIEF FRICTION

(RHU* friction) or: A few drops Juniper + Pine + Rosemary + Turpentine: 1–3 times a day.

– SLIMMING FRICTION

(MIN* friction) or: A few drops Juniper + Birth + Cypress + Geranium, as friction on legs, buttocks, tummy, arms twice a day.

– SLIMMING BATH

5 drops Juniper + 5 Geranium + 5 Cypress in 2 tablespoons green seaweed + 1 tablespoon sea water (or milk).

– WARMING UP MUSCLES

(VIT* friction) or: A few drops Juniper + Pine + Rosemary + Turpentine. Use before and after exercising.

My advice: essential oil of Juniper dissolves uric stones and residues, helps with elimination of kidney waste and slimming, of course. Hydrosol of Juniper can be an additional slimming, hygienic drink.

*See page 80.

Lavender – Lavendula officinalis
FOR SMALL CUTS AND CIRCULATION

– **Soothing, spasmodic, healing**.
– Insomnia, spasm, anxiety, migraine, all wounds: cuts, burns, insect bites, razor rash, acne, skin conditions.

Dosage
Internal use: 2–3 drops, 2–3 times a day on hand, in water or honey.
External use: A few drops diffused, as friction, or applied:
• to soothe children: on back of chest.
• for migraine: on temples.
• for anxiety   evening, on chest and back.
Treatment: Internal and external use for 1–3 weeks
Maintenance: 1 week a month or 3 weeks every 3 months.

Synergies – recipes
– INSOMNIA AND ANXIETY
Internal use: Lavender, Marjoram, Basil – 1 drop each at 5pm and before going to bed.
External use: Lavender friction + Marjoram: on chest, back and feet each evening. Bath: Lavender: each evening (3–5 drops).
– RESPIRATORY PROBLEMS
Internal use: Lavender + Pine + Eucalyptus: 1 drop of each twice daily.
– CHILDREN'S INSOMNIA
Internal use: Lavender + Orange, 1 drop each twice daily in water or honey.
– MIGRAINE
Friction: 15 drops Lavender and 3 Mint: on temples, forehead, nape and back: 2–3 times a day.
– RELAXATION
(NER* friction) or: Friction: Lavender + Marjoram + Rosewood + Petit grain + Lemongrass: a few drops at 5pm and before bedtime on solar plexus, neck, spine and soles of feet.
BATHS: in 2 tablespoons powdered milk or green seaweed:
• Lavender 10 drops, Rosewood 5 drops
• Lavender 10 drops, Marjoram 5 drops
• Lavender 10 drops, Orange 10 drops
• Lavender hydrosol: 1 tablespoon per bath for infants.
• Lavender essential oil is the only essential oil to be added undiluted to a bath.
Diffusion in atmosphere: all essential oils quoted under Relaxation, alone or mixed.
*See page 80.

– SKIN COMPOSITION: applied twice daily and/or vapour treatment
- Dry skin: Lavender + Rosewood + Rosemary or Rose.
- Oily skin: Lavender + Sage + Sassafras.
- Itchy skin: Lavender + Geranium and hydrosol of Lavender and Sage.
- Skin to heal: Lavender + Geranium + Rosemary + Rose.

– ALL TYPES OF WOUNDS, BURNS, RAZOR RASH, ACNE, SPOTS, HERPES, SCURF, MOUTH ULCERS: a few drops of Lavender on wound.

– TOILET WATER: 30ml Lavender in 250ml alcohol (70°).

My advice: Lavender is almost a panacea! It supplants alcohol and iodine, soothes, disinfects and heals children and adults.
It's the first essential oil in the natural pharmacy!
For babies: hydrosol of Lavender is remarkable!

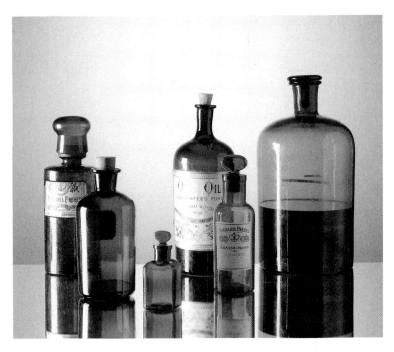

19th Cent. essential oil bottles.

Lemon – Citrus limonum
FOR WOMEN SLIMMING

– Reinforces natural immunities, tonic, general depurative and blood thinner.
– General fatigue, obesity, slimming, arteriosclerosis, wounds, herpes, acne, scurf, mouth ulcers.

Dosage
Internal use: 1–2 drops 3–5 times a day on hand, with water or honey.
External use: 3–5 drops on skin once or twice a day (all wounds, acne).
Treatment: Internal use twice daily for 3 weeks.
Prevention: 1 course of treatment each change of season.

Synergies – recipes
– SLIMMING
Internal use: Lemon + Juniper + Geranium – 1 drop each – twice daily in water or honey
+ external use = Caraway + Nutmeg – 5 drops each – as friction after meals on abdomen
+ internal use = Marjoram – 1 drop before bedtime, in water or honey
+ external use = friction with NER* or Lavender + Marjoram + Rosewood + Lemongrass + Petit grain, on chest, nape, spine (evening) and soles of feet and MIN† friction on 'round parts' (see Juniper).
– SPRING CURE
Internal use: 2 drops essential oil of Lemon 3 times a day + Juice of 3 lemons in 2 litres of water every day for 3 weeks.
– SKIN CARE
• Seborrhoea, oily skins = 2 drops Lemon + 2 Sassafras + 5 Lavender, applied twice a day.
• Regenerative mask (all skins) = 2 drops essential oil of Lemon + Water in 2 tablespoons of green clay.
– TOOTHPASTE = 2 drops of essential oil of Lemon + water + clay. Brush teeth and massage gums.
– oil for brittle nails = 10 drops essential oil of Lemon in a teaspoon of Wheat germ oil. Massage twice a week.
– PERFUMES
Lemon + Vervain or Lemon + Geranium or Lemon + Ylang-ylang 15ml in 100ml alcohol 70% + 1ml Clary Sage to fix the perfume.

*See page 80.

† See page 81.

– FRESH DRINKS
Lemon + Geranium or Lemon + Cedar or Lemon + Orange or Lemon +
Mint or Lemon + Rosemary.
• 1 drop each + honey + water + ice cubes. Serve as 'long drink'.
• 1 drop each + honey + warm water. Serve as 'tea'.
– CULINARY THERAPY
1–4 drops essential oil of Lemon in sorbet, flans, desserts, custards.

*My advice: it is a woman's No. 1 essential oil. Each of us should take a
cure of lemon (essential oil) + juice either for prevention or maintenance
once a year and make a habit of using essential oil in drinks instead of
cordials.*

Marjoram – Origanum marjorana
FOR ANXIETY

– **Balances neuro-vegetative nervous system, relaxes.**
Anxieties, depressive state, insomnia.

Dosage
Internal use: 1–2 drops twice a day on hand, in water or honey.
External use:
Friction: 10–20 drops, at 5pm and in the evening on chest and back.
Bath: 5 drops in 2 tablespoons of powdered milk or green seaweed.
Treatment: Internal and external use for 3 weeks.
Maintenance: 1–2 courses of treatment a year.

Synergies – recipes
– FRICTION (NER* friction)
Marjoram + Lavender + Rosewood + Petit grain + Lemongrass: twice daily
on solar plexus, nape of neck, spine and soles of feet.
– RELAXING BATH
5 drops Marjoram + 5 Lavender in 2 tablespoons of powdered milk or
green seaweed.
– COMPOSITION FOR DIFFUSER, SLEEP, RELAXATION
• Marjoram + Lavender + Pine + Rosewood + exotic Vervain.
• Marjoram + Lavender + Petit grain + Neroli.
• Marjoram + Lavender + Pine + exotic Vervain + Rosewood + Mint.
– FRICTION FOR 'MIGRAINE, SPASM'
A few drops of Marjoram or Marjoram + Chamomile + Lavender on
painful spot and solar plexus.
– RELAXING DRINK
At 5 pm and at bedtime: 2 drops Marjoram in warm water + honey.

*NOTE: 1 drop of Marjoram + 1 drop of Basil is a very specific remedy
against anxiety: take it 3–4 times a day + 1 NER friction twice daily.*

*My advice: even better results with Marjoram + Basil in a synergistic
blend. Internal and External treatment in all cases of exhaustion of
nervous system.*

*See page 80.

Mint – Mentha Vera or Piperata
FOR REJUVENATION

– Tonic, digestive and bactericidal.
General fatigue, impotence, bad breath, intestinal parasites.

Dosage
Internal use: 1 drop 1–3 times a day, after meals as digestive, or in morning as tonic in water or honey. No prolonged treatment (3–7 days only)
No external use
Maintenance: 1 week every 3 months

Synergies – recipes
– COMPOSITION FOR HOT FEET
15ml Lavender + 3 mint, a few drops as friction on feet morning and evening or before going dancing; it will refresh you!
– SLIMMING COMPOSITION
Rosemary, Birch, Cypress, Juniper, Lavender, Pine Mint (= CEL* friction). Friction twice daily on feet, legs, up to hips.
– BATH
Never use mint in baths! It freezes you!
– HYGIENIC DRINK
5 tablespoons of hydrosol of Mint per litre of water makes a cool drink suitable for adults and children.
– FOOT FRICTION with hydrosol of Mint: morning and evening and before getting up: relieves – refreshes.

Precautions:
Never use essential oil of Mint straight as a friction or in bath water, it would freeze you.
– Evening: essential oil of Mint is a light aphrodisiac and delays sleep.

*See page 81.

Nutmeg – Myristica fragrans
FOR A TONIC

– General cerebral stimulant, digestive, aphrodisiac.
Intellectual fatigue, impotence, flatulence...

Dosage
Internal use: 1–2 drops after meals (preferably Caraway + Nutmeg) on hand.
External use: see synergies.
Maintenance: Once or twice a year for three weeks.

Synergies – recipes
– STIMULATING AND APHRODISIAC FRICTION (VIT* friction) or:
A few drops Nutmeg + Rosemary + Savory Geranium + Lavender + Coriander + Pine, morning and evening, as friction on chest, back, soles of feet.
– DIGESTIVE FRICTION (DIG* friction) or
Caraway 10 drops + 10 drops Nutmeg: as friction on abdomen after meals.
– TONIC BATH FOR NERVOUS SYSTEM
5 drops Nutmeg + 5 Lavender + Marjoram, in 2 tablespoons of sea water.
– PERFUME
In a foundation, essential oil of Nutmeg imparts a masculine strength to a soft, flowery fragrance.
– COOKERY
1–3 drops when serving starchy dishes.

NOTE: Essential oils of Nutmeg and Coriander are 'sister' – tonic, physical sensual and intellectual.

*See page 80.

Orange – Neroli – Petit Grain –
Citrus vulgaris / aurantium / cinensis
FOR INSOMNIA

– Nervous sedative No. 1.
Tranquilizer for children, slightly hypnotic, tonicardiac, bactericidal.

Dosage
Internal use:
Orange: 3–5 drops at 5pm and bedtime on hand, in water or honey.
Petit grain: 1–2 drops at 5pm and at bedtime.
Neroli: ½ to 1 drop at 5pm and at bedtime.
External use: friction with 15–20 drops orange, on chest and back before bedtime.
Apply a few drops, morning and evening, on skin to regenerate.
Treatment: twice daily for 1–3 weeks.
Maintenance: according to needs.

Synergies – recipes
– SEDATIVE FRICTIONS
15ml Orange + 2 Petit grain + 1 Neroli, for adults.
Lavender, Marjoram, Rosewood, Petit grain, Lemongrass = NER* friction.
20–30 drops of mixture twice in the evening.
– SEDATIVE BATH
5 drops Orange + 2 Petit grain + 5 Lavender in 2 tablespoons of milk or green seaweed.
– POWERFUL SEDATIVE BATH
1 drop of Neroli + 2 Petit grain + 5 Marjoram in 2 tablespoons of powdered milk or green seaweed.
– COMPOSITION FOR DIFFUSER
• Lavender + Petit grain + Pine.
• Lavender + Petit grain + Neroli + Marjoram.
– PERFUME (A very Egyptian aroma)
100ml alcohol (70°C) + 15ml Petit grain + 1 drop Neroli.
– COOKERY
3–5 drops Orange in flans, desserts or cakes.

NOTE: Essential oil of Orange is obtained by expressing the fresh zest of sweet oranges. Essential oil of Petit grain is obtained by expressing the leaves of Seville oranges. Essential oil of Neroli is obtained by distilling the flowers of sweet oranges.

* see page 80

Oregano – *Origanum vulgare*
ANTISEPTIC

– Antiseptic, tonic for nervous system.
All infectious problems, fatigue. Best avoided in pregnancy.

Dosage
Internal use: 1 drop 3 times a day on hand, in water or honey.
External use: frictions always diluted in other others.
Treatment: 3 times a day for 3 weeks.
Prevention: 1 week every 3 months.

Synergies – recipes
– TONIC 'ANTI-FLU' TODDY
1 drop Oregano + 1 Thyme + 1 Cinnamon + 1 Clove + 1 Geranium
+ 1 Ginger (optional) in lemon juice + honey + warm water.
– 'INDIGESTION' DRINK
1 drop Oregano + 1 Clove + 1 Ginger + 1 honey + warm water after meals.
– 'TONIC' FRICTION, FLU, CHILLS, FATIGUE (=VIT* friction)
5ml Oregano + 5 Marjoram + 5 Vervain + 5 Basil + 5 Lavender – a few
drops twice daily on chest, back, soles of feet.
– 'ANTI-CELLULITE' FRICTION (CEL Friction)
A few drops Oregano + Birch + Rosemary + Cypress + Geranium +
Lavender + Pine + Mint (CEL* friction) morning and evening on legs,
buttocks, stomach or CEL* friction + 108* friction.
– DISINFECTING COMPOSITION FOR ATMOSPHERE
15ml Oregano + 30ml Lavender + 30ml Geranium + 20ml exotic Vervain
+ 5ml Neroli or Cinnamon or Sandalwood.
– COMPOSITION FOR BURNS, SEPTIC WOUNDS
6ml Oregano + 8 Lavender + 6 Geranium.
A few drops on skin every 3 hours or as compress.
NOTE 1:
• *Essential oil of Oregano is the best antiseptic essential oil.*
• *Hydrosol of Oregano offers all its tonic and anti-fatigue properties*
when used as a daily drink: 2 soup spoons in a litre and a half of water,
daily.
NOTE 2:
It is the No. 1 essential oil of the aromatogram. Essential oil of Oregano
can stop and kill Koch's bacillus: the Mycobacterium tuberculosis,
causative organism of tuberculosis, thyphus in less than 4 hours!
(Experiments by Dr Valnet.).

* See page 81.

Pine – Pinus sylvestris
FOR COUGHS

– Antiseptic for respiratory tubes
Complaints of the respiratory tubes (colds, tracheal catarrh, pneumonia, asthma, flu...)

Dosage
Internal use: 1–3 drops 3 times a day on hand, in water or honey.
External use: friction and inhalation of 20–30 drops Pine in bowl of warm water and inhale for 3–5 minutes. Use in an aroma diffuser, too.
Treatment: twice daily for 3 weeks.
Prevention: 1 course of treatment before winter.

Synergies – recipes
– 'ANTI-COUGH' TODDY
1 drop Pine + Eucalyptus + juice of 1 orange + juice of 1 lemon + hot water + honey 2–3 times a day.
– SOOTHING COUGH FRICTIONS
• Pine/Eucalyptus + Oregano + Lavender: a few drops of each.
• Pine + Eucalyptus: a few drops of each.
– SCABS
Apply some drops of 15ml Lavender + 5 Pine + 5 Eucalyptus + 5 Sage twice daily.
– HEALTH DRINK FOR CHILDREN: soothing
1 teaspoon hydrosol of Pine in 1 cup of warm water + honey or 2 tablespoons in a litre of cold water + honey or fructose.
– INFANTS' FRICTION (chills)
Hydrosol of Pine on chest and back, together with hydrosol of Lavender (for very young babies).
– COMPOSITION FOR DIFFUSION
• Essential oil of Pine or Pine + Lavender or see Eucalyptus.
• Essential oil of Fir, Pine, Mandarin and Orange: very acceptable to children.
• Essential oil of Pine + Thyme + Eucalyptus.
• Essential oil of Pine + Fir + Sandalwood + Cedarwood.

Rose / Rosewood – Rosa / Aniba rosaeaodora
FOR THE SKIN

– Strong issue regenerator
Anti-wrinkle, dermatitis and skin fatigue.

Dosage
Applied: 4–5 drops of Rosewood essential oil once or twice a day on cleansed skin as treatment for 3–6 weeks.
Baths: 10 drops in 2 tablespoons powdered milk or green seaweed mixed in bath water.
Treatment: 6 weeks.
Prevention: 3–4 times a year for 3 weeks.

Synergies – recipes
– SPECIAL 'ANTI-WRINKLE' BODY OIL
100ml Wheat germ oil + 15 Rosewood + 1 Rose
– SPECIAL FACE OIL
80ml Wheat germ oil + 20 St John's Wort oil + 15 Rosewood + 1 Rose.
– FIRMING UP OIL: the perfect "rejuvenating" oil.
100ml Wheat germ oil + 10 Rosewood + 10 Rosemary + 1 Rose.
– SOOTHING BATHS (see dosage)
5 drops Rosewood + 5 Lavender or Cedar.
– VAPOUR TREATMENT AFTER MASKS
• Dry skin: Lavender + Rosewood + Rose Geranium.
• Oily skin: Lavender + Rosewood + Lemon.
• Wrinkled skin: Rosewood + Rosemary + Sandalwood.
• Itchy skin: Rosewood + Lavender + Chamomile.
– SCENTED MILKS 'AFTER BATH, AFTER SUN'
• Geranium: 250ml of neutral body milk + 10 Rosewood + 10 Geranium.
• Rose: 250ml of neutral body milk + 10ml Rosewood + 5 drops Rose.
– TOILET WATER
250ml alcohol (70°C) + Rosewood + 1 Rose.
– TOILET PERFUME
100ml alcohol (70°C) + Rosewood + 10 drops Rose.
– AROMATIC BODY OILS (ABO; the very special oils of Nelly Grosjean)
In a base of Wheat germ oil and St John's Wort oil, Rosewood and essential oil of Rose (see face oil) for 100ml add:
5ml essential oil of Mint = ABO fresh
15ml essential oil of Rosemary = ABO tonic
10ml essential oil of Geranium = ABO comfort
5ml essential oil of Neroli = ABO relax.
NOTE: Each time you use Rose, mix 10 drops of Rosewood essential oil with 1 drop of Rose essential oil: much easier to use.
Remember that essential oil of Rose is one of the most rejuvenating oils.

Sage - *Salvia officinalis*
FOR GYNAECOLOGICAL PROBLEMS

– Anti-perspiration, hypotensive, anti lacteal

General, menopausal fatigue, prevents hot flushes, regulator of menstruation, eliminates excessive perspiration (armpits, feet), hair care, seborrhoea, itching, thinning hair... dries up lactation.

Dosage

Internal use: 1–3 drops daily between meals licked from hand, in water or honey.

External use: friction twice daily.

Treatment: 1 drop twice daily for a week.

Maintenance: 1 course of treatment every 3 months.

Synergies - recipes

– FRICTIONS, MASSAGES

• Feet: 15ml Sage + 10 Lavender twice daily on feet.

• Hot feet: 15ml Sage + 10 Cypress + 10 Lavender + 1 Mint twice daily.

– HAIR CARE

10ml Sage + 15 Lavender + 5 Thyme. 100 drops on scalp once a week, on the day before shampooing for 6 weeks. Eliminates seborrhoea, itching... helps with regrowth, beautifies tired hair.

– SUPER REVITALISING FORMULA

15ml Sage + 15 Cedar + 15 Lavender + 5 Thyme + 1 Ylang-ylang. 100 drops twice weekly or 50 drops twice weekly for 6 weeks, then once a month.

On day before washing, apply to scalp and leave overnight.

– 'HEAVY' CONGESTED LEGS FORMULA

15ml Sage + 15 Cypress + 3 Mint. 30–40 drops twice daily from soles of feet to knee + rotating ankle exercises + sleep with propped up legs (10 to 15cms).

– WARM SPRAY AFTER FACE CARE

5 drops Sage + 5 Juniper + 5 Lavender. Disinfects and softens.

– BATHS

• Anti-rheumatic: 3 drops Sage + 3 Lavender + 2 Marjoram in 2 tablespoons sea water (or milk).

• Heavy legs: 5 drops Sage + 5 Cypress + 10 Lavender in 2 tablespoons green seaweed.

– PERFUME

To the composition of all perfumes and toilet waters, add a few drops of essential oil of Clary sage as a 'fixative' to perfume.

Special note for hydrosol of Sage: Most women would have to have 3 or 4 courses a year of hydrosol of Sage with 2 tablespoons per litre and a half of water for 3 weeks. It is especially recommended for all circulatory problems, and also for gynological problems, too.

Sassafras – *Sassafras albidum*
ANTI-TOBACCO

– Encourages perspiration, pain killer, skin disinfectant, diuretic
Tobacco antidote, skin care for acne, ordinary stings or poisonous bites...

Dosage
Internal use: 1–3 drops 3 times a day in water or honey.
External use: a few drops, morning and evening, applied to skin to
regenerate or disinfect.
8–10 drops every two hours, on stings and poisonous bites.

Synergies – recipes
– ANTI-TOBACCO COCKTAIL
1 drop Sassafras + 1 Sage + 1 Geranium + 1 Marjoram + 1 Lavender + hot
water + honey + 1 hydrosol of Mint or Mint cordial. Serve with ice.
– VERY EFFICIENT ANTI-TOBACCO TREATMENT
• 2–4 'anti-tobacco cocktails' daily
• 2 frictions a day of same mixture on solar plexus, back, nape of neck,
spine and soles of feet
• diffusion in atmosphere of mixture exotic Vervain + Rosegeranium +
Pine + Cedar + Mint in equal parts to breathe all night or at least 3 hours
a day.
– VAPOUR TREATMENTS
2–3 drops Sassafras + Juniper + Turpentine once a day and before care of
clogged skin
3 drops Sassafras + 6 Lavender in 2 teaspoons of cold honey. Apply to 5–8
minutes. Remove with warm water.
– SOLUTION TO DISINFECT SKIN
15ml Sassafras + 15 Carrot + 15 Lavender, applied morning and evening,
5–7 drops alternatively with 15ml Rosewood and 10 drops of Rose or
Rosemary for skins to be regenerated... + spraying with hydrosol of Cedar.

Vervain – Verbena officinalis
FOR RELAXATION AND HAPPINESS

– Regulates neuro-vegetative system, tonifies heart, renders harmonious and creative.
Fatigue, disorders of the nervous system, antidote for snakes' venom.

Dosage
Internal use: 1–2 drops 2–3 times a day on hand or in honey.
External use: 10–20 drops of Vervain: always diluted in Wheat germ oil or essential oil of Lavender.
No friction, no bath with undiluted essential oil of Vervain.
Diffusion in atmosphere: the essential oil everyone loves, under all circumstances: exotic Vervain; which is a mix of 3 Vervain varieties formulated by Nelly Grosjean.
Treatment: Twice a day for 3 weeks.
Maintenance: 1 week a month or every 3 months.

Synergies – recipes
– MORNING TONIC FRICTION
5ml Vervain + Geranium + 5 Lemon, a few drops in morning after cool shower, on chest, solar plexus, nape of neck, back and soles of feet.
– EVENING REGENERATIVE FRICTION
5ml Vervain + 5 Lavender + 5 Marjoram + 5 Lemongrass, a few drops after hot bath or before bedtime.
– DIFFUSION IN ATMOSPHERE
• Pleasant: Exotic Vervain + Lemongrass.
• Good temper: Exotic Vervain + Rosewood.
• Anti-tobacco: Exotic Vervain + Geranium.
• Ideal: Exotic Vervain.

NOTE 1: The Vervain infusion helps with lactation and childbirth. To take as treatment at the end of pregnancy.
NOTE 2: Internal use and friction: medicinal Vervain. Diffusion: exotic Vervain.

"Exotic Vervain is my own special oil – my 'oil of happiness' and 'bonheur'; a mixture of 3 different vervains."

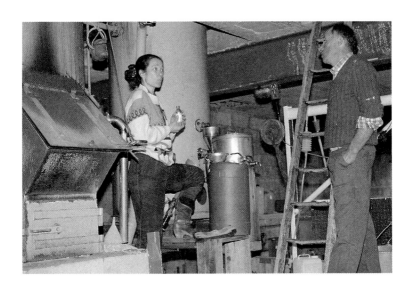

Nelly Grosjean choosing essences with her private distiller.

CHAPTER 2

Therapy

Charts and Classifications

- Common Problems

- Main Properties

- Put Together Your Own Natural Pharmacy

- Summary Chart

- Classification by Illness

- Classification by Plants

Common Problems

> *How would you be able to stand upright*
> *if an invisible hand did not support you* The Koran

Digestive system

Flatulence: Caraway + Nutmeg and DIG* friction.
Colitis: Cinnamon + DIG* friction.
Constipation: No essential oil: treatment with fresh
                vegetable juice + food supplements, exercise and
                relaxation.

Additional advice:
– eat fruit between meals.
– avoid wrong combinations.
– chew well and take time to eat quietly.
– watch for good intestinal elimination.
– + laxative infusion + eat cooked vegetables, toasted bran or wholemeal
  bread.
– fresh vegetable juice or milk-fermented juices as aperitif.
– a daily health drink with hydrosol of Sage, Rosemary, Oregano...

Circulatory problems

Thick blood: Lemon + 108*.
Heavy legs: Cypress + Lemon, CEL* friction and 108* friction.
Piles: Cypress + Lavender + a treatment of 108* friction.

Additional advice:
– eat raw food + spices + garlic, onion...
– drink a lot of water between meals.
– exercise.
– avoid starch, sugar and animal fat.
– eat less red meat.
– drink vegetable juice before meals.
– course of hydrosol of Sage, Juniper, Elder...
*See page 81.

Cellulite

Cypress + Juniper + Lemon (external use) or
Cypress + Juniper + Birch + Turpentine or CEL* + 108* frictions (external use).

Additional advice:
– conscious breathing.
– relaxation and sleep.
– see 'circulatory' advice: " cellulite arises from a circulatory problem and a lack of relaxation" [†]

Gynaecological problems

Amenorrhea:	Sage + 108* friction + course of hydrosol of Clarified Sage.
Dysmenorrhoea:	Same.
Painful periods:	Same.
Leucorrhea:	Lavender douche.

Additional advice:
– Strengthen the abdomen (breathing exercises).
– Regulate food patterns.
– Sexual harmony and mental equilibrium.
– Learn to understand psychological disorders which generally occur around menstruation.
– Need to discover the causes of disturbance, cleansing the body...
– Course of hydrosol of Sage, Pine or Oregano.

Rheumatism

Juniper external + RHU[‡] friction for relief of pain.

Additional advice:
– Cut down or totally avoid animal proteins during treatment (especially cheese).
– Drink large amounts of water or diuretic infusions (Birch, Meadowsweet, Horsetail...)
– Course of hydrosol of Fennel, Pine, Thyme, Celery, Juniper, Elder.

---

*See page 81.
[†]Refer to *Aromatherapie 2, des huiles essentielles pour votre santé* by the same author.
Frictions made by Nelly Grosjean are by mail order only from VIE AROME.
See address on last page.
[‡]See page 80.

Respiratory problems

Cold, Flu   Eucalyptus + diffusion with Respiratory + RES* friction
                   + hydrosol of Pine, Thyme, Hyssop, Eucalyptus.

Additional advice:
– Breathing exercises.
– Expand your rib cage.
– Control your breathing.
– Clean air and exercise.
– Diet: cut out sweets and starches.
– Importance of nasal hygiene. (Works by L. and B. de Bardo)

Nervous System

Insomnia: Marjoram + Lavender or Orange
                   + diffused Lavender or relaxing composition
                   + relaxing bath with aromatic oils (ABO relax[†])
                   + relaxing NER* friction.
Anxiety: Marjoram + Basil: nutrition of the nervous cells
                   + exotic Vervain (diffused)
                   + NER* or HAR[†] friction.
Tiredness: Rosemary + Savory (internal)
                   + VIT* friction + diffused tonic composition.
Lack of energy: Morning VIT* or APH* friction
(sexual, mental,   + Rosemary (internal) + hydrosol of Rosemary,
physical)   Savory, Oregano.

Additional advice:
Raw food + trace elements + mineral salts (multi-minerals and specialities)
+ Wheat germ oil + raw vegetable juice.
– Importance of good breathing (essential oil diffusion + ionisation).
– Importance of conscious relaxation.
– Physical exercise and clean air + relaxation.
– Cut out all stimulants (tobacco, alcohol, coffee, sugar, tea).
The nervous system consumes 14 times more oxygen than any other living cell.
– Balanced nutrition, first-class food.
– Recovery through sleep (hours before midnight count double).
– Course of hydrosol of Marjoram, Oregano, Savory, Rosemary in rotation.

*See page 80.

[†]See page 81.

Skin

"Skin, mirror of your health." (Dr Ribollet)

Dry skin: Rose + Rosewood + hydrosol of Rosemary and Lavender
                  and Clarified sage or Wild Rose.
Wrinkled skin: Rose and Rosemary + hydrosol of Rosemary and
                  Lavender and Chamomile.
Greasy skin: Rose + Sassafras + hydrosol of Cedar and Lavender.

Additional advice:
– Draining of liver and intestinal elimination.
– Add a course of B group vitamins.
– Course of Wheat germ oil (1 teaspoon a day), vitamin E.
– Specific treatment with aromatic oils.
– Regular spraying with hydrosols of Rose, Sage, Lavender, Rosemary,
Cedar, Chamomile...

Hair

All problems   106* friction = Sage + Thyme + Lavender + Ylang-ylang
                  + lotion of Hydrosol of Wild Sage, Cedar, Thyme and
                  Lavender.

Additional advice:
– Freeze-dried yeast (B vitamins).
– Draining of liver (black radish and artichoke).
– Specific treatment with Essential Oils.
– A very high proportion of raw food, raw vegetable juice before meals.

Sexual Problems[†]

Muscle tone: See tiredness
Frigidity/Impotence: + general cleansing necessary and personal
                      compositions of revitalisation or APH[‡] friction +
                      hydrosol of Savory and Oregano.

Additional advice:
– Important to know how to conduct a harmonious sexual life.
– Exercise and fresh air.
– Balanced nutrition (+ vegetable juices + food supplements).
– Relaxation.
– In all cases, this advice is to be followed in additional to the
recommendations for a good, hygienic lifestyle.

---

*Frictions made by Vie Arôme. See page 81.
†Refer to *Aromatherapie 2, des huiles essentielles pour votre sante*, by the same author.
Frictions made by Nelly Grosjean are by mail order only from VIE AROME.
‡See page 80.

Table of Essential Oils: Main properties

MAIN PROPERTIES	ESSENTIAL OILS
Antibiotics	**Oregano** No. 1 for antiseptic properties, **Cinnamon, Thyme, Clove, Savory.** Cajuput, Pine, Lavender.
Anti-perspiration	**Sage.**
Antiseptics	
– Intestinal	**Caraway, Cinnamon.** Eucalyptus. **Thyme.** Bergamot, Oregano, Nutmeg.
– Genito-urinary	**Sandalwood, Ylang-ylang.** Cedar, Hyssop.
– Pulmonary/ Respiratory	**Cajuput, Thyme, Oregano.** Niaouli, Pine, Rosemary.
Anti-spasmodics	**Chamomile.** Bergamot, Tarragon, Basil.
Anti-tobacco	**Sassafras.** Rosegeranium, Marjoram, Lavender.
Anti-wrinkles	**Rose, Rosewood, Rosemary.** Sandalwood, Ylang-ylang.
Aphrodisiac	**Cinnamon, Ginger, Rosemary, Savory, Ylang ylang.** Nutmeg, Coriander, Sandalwood, Clove, Rosewood, see Ginger.
Digestive	**Caraway, Nutmeg, Coriander, Cumin, Mint.** Tarragon, Basil, Rosemary.
Diuretic	**Lemon, Birch, Juniper, Sandalwood**, Cedar.
Pain Killers	**Lavender, Marjoram, Chamomile, Clove** (teeth). Cajuput. See Juniper.
Respiratory	**Eucalyptus, Pine, Thyme, Hyssop.** Cajuput, Niaouli.
Revitalising	
– Intellect	**Coriander.** Tarragon, Clove, Rosemary. See Rosemary.
– Glandular system	**Sandalwood, Savory, Ylang-ylang, Rosemary, Cinnamon.**
– General state	**Rosemary, Savory, Oregano.** Coriander.
– Sexual function	See Aphrodisiac.
– Nervous system	**Basil + Marjoram.** Vervain.

MAIN PROPERTIES	ESSENTIAL OILS
Scar healers	**Lavender, Rosegeranium, Rosemary**. Rosewood, Sandalwood.
Slimming	Lemon, Juniper, Rose, Geranium, Birch (see Juniper for baths and slimming frictions).
Soothing	See pain killers.
– Pain	Lavender, Marjoram, Neroli. Orange, Petit grain.
– Relaxation	Marjoram, Lavender. Chamomile.
– Anti-depressant	Basil + Marjoram. Vervain.
Essential oil from the aromatogram	Oregano, Savory, Cinnamon, Thyme. Clove, Cajuput, Pine, Lavender.

(Oils especially effective for this purpose are highlighted in bold.)

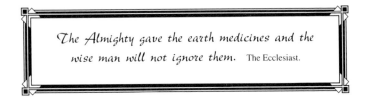

The Almighty gave the earth medicines and the wise man will not ignore them.   The Ecclesiast.

Put Together Your Own 'Natural Pharmacy'.

Green Clay (tube):
Any wound, sting, burn, cut, scratch... brings out foreign bodies, splinters, pus... heals scar tissue.

Chloride of magnesium:
For any infection, prepare 1 litre of water with 20 grams of chloride of magnesium. Take 2 tablespoons twice daily, or every 3 hours.

Essential oils of Lavender or Rosegeranium: heals, soothes.
On all wounds, stings, burns, small cuts, razor rash, cuts... Can also be used with a clay poultice.

Essential oil of Mint: Digestive, refreshing. 1 or 2 drops after meals.

Essential oil of Caraway + Nutmeg: strong digestive (or DIG* friction) 2 or 3 drops after meals + 20 drops friction on abdomen, after meals, in case of wind, flatulence...

Essential oil of Lemon: General antiseptic. 2 or 3 drops applied on erupting spots, herpes, impetigo several times a day.

Essential oil of Sage: Anti-perspirant.
A few drops applied on armpits and feet avoid unpleasant perspiration (108* friction). 1 drop in water or honey 3 times a day to ease painful menstruation + CEL* friction at the base of stomach.

Essential oil of Rosemary or Oregano or Thyme: powerful antibiotic and antiseptic.
A drop (of either) 3–5 times a day in case of biological disorders of viral or microbial origin (angina, asthma, hepatitis, chills...)

*See page 81.

Essential oil of Eucalyptus: pulmonary and respiratory, antiseptic.
1–3 drops 3 times a day + friction chest and back + aroma diffusion to prevent flu... RES* friction involves both friction, inhalation and internal treatment.

Essential oils of Juniper + Pine + Rosemary + Turpentine or (RHU* friction).
Instantly soothes any pain: rheumatism, rheumatoid arthritis, osteoarthritis, muscles... also warms up before exercise.

Essential oil of Cinnamon: intestinal antiseptic.
1 drop 2 or 3 times every 2 hours stops diarrhoea in less than 4 hours.

Essential oil of Chamomile: antispasmodic
1–2 drops 3 times a day + friction on temples and around nose, soothes sinusitis.

Essential oils of Marjoram + Lavender or NER* friction: calming, relaxing.
A few drops as a friction on temples and base of neck to cure headaches... and encourage sleep.

Essential oil of Orange or Lavender: sedative for children.
1 drop Orange on 1 teaspoon of honey before going to bed + friction on chest and back with Orange + Lavender, makes children sleep.

Oil of St John's Wort – Our grandmother's 'red oil': for sunburn, burns, soothes and heals.
To be applied on neck and spine. According to Dr Breuss, a German doctor from early this century who used to treat with oil of St John's Wort and a course of vegetable juices, this oil has the particular effect of '"re-inflating" intervertebral cartilages'.

Summary Chart: Directions for Use and General Dosage

Dosage	Use	Treatment	Blend
DIFFUSION Aroma diffuser	In atmosphere	Once daily of diffusion	15ml for one week
FRICTIONS	On body	3 weeks to 3 months	20–50 drops blend. Use 1–3 times a day
INTERNAL USE	By mouth	1–3 weeks when necessary	1–3 drops 3 times a day
INHALATIONS	Vaporiser		3–10 drops in vaporiser
BATHS	Health baths and showers	Crisis 1–2 baths a day	3–10 drops per bath
VAPOUR TREATMENT	Skin	Prevention once a week	3–10 drops per bowl
MASKS	Skin	1–2 a week	1–5 drops per mask
MILKS	Skin and body	Daily	15ml in 250ml milk
BEAUTY FRICTIONS	Skin	3 weeks twice daily	3–5 drops blend
FEET	Feet	Daily 1–2 frictions	10–20 drops blend
HAIR FRICTIONS	Hair	6 weeks	50–100 drops 1 to 2 times a week
MASSAGE OILS	Body	Daily	15–30ml in 100ml oil
BEAUTY OILS	Face	For 3 weeks 3–4 times a year	5–15 drops 2 times a day
PERFUME	Perfume Toilet water		15ml in 100ml alcohol 70°C

Precautions: please refer to recipes given in the Quick Reference to Everyday Oils for Home Use.

Classification by Illness

Illness	Corresponding essential oils
Acne	LEMON, SASSAFRAS, Eucalyptus. See Skin and Cajuput oil.
Acne rosacea	CYPRESS, ROSEWOOD.
Ageing	LEMON. (See longevity)
Allergy	CHAMOMILE. Cedar, Rosewood, Lavender.
Alopecia	See Hair.
Amenorrhea	PARSLEY, LEMON, NUTMEG. Cypress, Sage, Geranium.
Angina	LEMON, SAVORY, OREGANO. Rose Geranium, Chamomile.
Anguish, Anxiety	BASIL + MARJORAM. See antidepressant and Lavender.
Anti-wrinkle	ROSE, ROSEWOOD, ROSEMARY.
Armpits	See anti-perspiration.
Asthma	HYSSOP. Lavender, Chamomile, Cajuput, Eucalyptus.
Bandages	Clay powder + LAVENDER + ROSEMARY + ROSEGERANIUM.
Biliary lithiasis	See gallstones.
Blisters	LAVENDER.
Boils	LAVENDER + LEMON.
Breath (halitosis)	MINT. Nutmeg.
Breasts (sore)	See chafing.
Bronchitis	HYSSOP, NIAOULI, CAJUPUT. See essential oil for respiratory problems.
Burns	LAVENDER + ROSEGERANIUM. Niaouli.
Cancer (prevention)	ONION. ROSE.
Cellulite	BIRCH, JUNIPER, CYPRESS, Oregano, Lavender, Rosemary.
Chafing	Lemon juice + essential oil of LAVENDER.
Chilblains	LAVENDER + Lemon juice.
Childbirth (to help)	Vervain infusion + Sage essential oil.
Cholera	MINT, OREGANO, THYME.
Cholesterol (excess)	ROSEMARY + ROSEGERANIUM.
Circulation	LEMON, CYPRESS, SAGE. See essential oil for circulation.
Cirrhosis	OREGANO, ROSEMARY.
Cold	
– Simple cold	All essential oils for respiratory problems.
– Hay fever	Chamomile, Lavender, Hyssop.

Illness	Corresponding essential oils
Colonbacillosis	OREGANO. Oregano No. 1 for antiseptic properties.
Colic	CINNAMON. Caraway.
Conjunctivitis	<u>Juice of lemon.</u> See Lemon recipe.
Constipation	*Plants, a balanced diet, but no specific essential oil for constipation.*
Corpulence	See Slimming.
Cough – Tracheitis	PINE + EUCALYPTUS + coated pills (clay).
Crevices (body)	LAVENDER + LEMON. Rosewood.
Cuts	LAVENDER. See wounds.
Cystitis	CAJUPUT OIL, SANDALWOOD. Lavender.
Dental	
– abscess	CLOVE. See Teeth.
– cavities	CLOVE. Lavender.
– toothache	Children: CHAMOMILE.
Dermatitis	See Skin.
Diabetes	JUNIPER, EUCALYPTUS, LEMON + Robert Geranium (plant).
Diarrhoea/Dysentery	CINNAMON. Caraway.
Digestion	See Digestive system.
Distention	See Flatulence and digestive system.
Dysmenorrhoea	SAGE, CYPRESS. Tarragon.
Dyspepsia	See Digestive system.
Emopytysis	LEMON, EUCALYPTUS, CHAMOMILE.
Enterocolitis	LAVENDER, CARAWAY. Chamomile.
Epidemics (prevention)	See Antiseptics, Antibiotics (mainly diffused in atmosphere).
Excitement	See Soothers.
Eczema	ROSE. Lavender, Rosegeranium, Juniper, Sandalwood.
Fatigue	*Fatigue or the exhaustion of vital energies necessitates revising the life style: balanced diet, exercise, deep breathing, fresh air, relaxation, positive thinking, harmony.*
– General	LEMON, ROSEGERANIUM. Rosemary, Oregano.
– Physical	ROSEMARY, CORIANDER. Oregano.
– Nervous	BASIL + MARJORAM. Lavender.
– Intellectual	CORIANDER, CLOVE, ROSEMARY, Rosewood + Cinnamon + Chamomile + diffusion in the atmosphere of Tonic blend.

Illness	Corresponding essential oils
– Sexual	CINNAMON, GINGER, NUTMEG, CORIANDER, SAVORY, Rosemary, Sandalwood, Ylang-ylang.
– Moral	<u>Exotic Vervain in diffusion + HAR* frictions.</u> See Anti-depressant.
– Muscular	ROSEMARY + Juniper, Turpentine.
Fevers	LEMON + SAGE.
Flatulence	CARAWAY. NUTMEG. Coriander, Cumin.
Flu	EUCALYPTUS, THYME. Oregano, Cinnamon. See Cinnamon for anti-flu toddy.
Feet	
– Hot	LAVENDER + MINT + ROSEMARY + Rosewood + Rosegeranium. See Cypress recipe.
– Sweaty	SAGE + CYPRESS + LAVENDER.
Gonorrhea	Sandalwood, Thuja, Savory.
Gout	JUNIPER. Cajuput, Rosemary.
Gums	
– To strengthen	LEMON
– Gingivitis	LEMON + powdered clay.
Hair	
– Loss	LAVENDER + SAGE + THYME.
– Improvement	YLANG-YLANG, CEDAR. Lavender, Sage, Thyme.
– Greasy	LAVENDER + SAGE + THYME + CEDAR.
Headaches	LAVENDER, CHAMOMILE.
Head Cold	See Cold.
Healing	LAVENDER + ROSEGERANIUM, Rosemary, Niaouli.
Heart Palpitations	PETIT GRAIN, NEROLI. Mint.
Herpes	LEMON, ROSE GERANIUM, OREGANO.
Hiccups	TARRAGON.
Hypertension	LEMON.
Hypotension	HYSSOP.
Hysteria	NEROLI. Lavender, Marjoram.
Heavy Legs	CYPRESS + SAGE + Mint + Rosegeranium.
Impotence	See Aphrodisiacs.
Indigestion	See Digestive System and Clove recipe.
Infections	See Antiseptics.
Insect Bites	LAVENDER + ROSEGERANIUM + CINNAMON. See Cinnamon recipe.
Insomnia	
– Children	LAVENDER, ORANGE.

Illness	Corresponding essential oils
– Adults	LAVENDER, MARJORAM. Petit grain, Neroli, Orange.
Intestinal problems	See Digestive and Antiseptics: intestinal. CARAWAY 'No. 1 intestinal oxygeniser'.
Irritability	BASIL + MARJORAM. NEROLI + ORANGE. LAVENDER.
Jaundice	OREGANO, ROSEMARY, LEMON.
Laryngitis	LAVENDER + PINE + CAJUPUT.
Leucorrhea	SANDALWOOD + LAVENDER. Juniper. Hyssop.
Lice	ROSEGERANIUM. Lavender, Sage
Liver (deficiency)	ROSEMARY, MINT.
Longevity	*Healthy diet, exercise, deep breathing and regular use of essential oils as frictions and in diffusion, and positive thinking are all factors for good health and longevity.*
Loss of strength	See Fatigue.
Malaria	OREGANO, THYME, CINNAMON, Savory.
Melancholia	See Revitalizing.
Menopause	SAGE. Cypress, Lemon.
Migraine	LAVENDER, CHAMOMILE, MINT. Marjoram. See Lavender recipe.
Menstruation and female problems	See Amenorrhea. Dysmenorrhoea. Leucorrhea.
Mental instability	BASIL + MARJORAM. BERGAMOT.
Mouth ulcer	Lemon.
Mumps	CHAMOMILE (external). Lemon juice. See Lemon recipe.
Muscles	ROSEWOOD, LAVENDER, SAGE. Savory.
Mycoses (feet)	LAVENDER + SAGE + ROSE + ROSEWOOD.
Nausea	ROSEMARY, TARRAGON, MINT. See Clove recipe.
Nephritis	SANDALWOOD, YLANG-YLANG, JUNIPER.
Nervous breakdown	BASIL + MARJORAM. See Anti-depressant.
Neurasthenia	See Anti-depressant.
Nicotine addiction:	SASSAFRAS. Rosegeranium, Marjoram.
Nocturnal perspiration	SAGE.
Obesity	JUNIPER, LEMON. See Slimming. Recipe: Lemon or Juniper or Rosegeranium.
Osteoarthritis	See Anti-rheumatism.

Illness	Corresponding essential oils
Otitis	<u>Juice of lemon.</u> See Lemon recipe.
Oxyuris	GARLIC (essential oil diluted 2%). OREGANO, CARAWAY, MINT.
Pains	See Pain killers.
Papillome/mild tumour	THUJA (external).
Paralysis (after effects)	*ALL ESSENTIAL OILS in friction or in diffusion in the atmosphere to regenerate the whole body.*
Perspiration	
– Excessive	SAGE + CYPRESS + LAVENDER + ROSEWOOD + MINT.
– Feet	SAGE, CYPRESS, LAVENDER. See Hot Feet.
Piles	LAVENDER + CYPRESS (external).
Pneumonia	See Respiratory problems.
Prostate	THUJA, SANDALWOOD.
Pruritis	LAVENDER.
Psoriasis	See Cajuput.
Rhinitis	LAVENDER, CHAMOMILE.
Rheumatism	JUNIPER + Pine + Turpentine + Rosemary + Eucalyptus.
Seasickness	MINT.
Scabies	See Pine recipe.
Scabs	See Lavender recipe.
Scurf	LEMON. Rosegeranium.
Seborrhoea	
– Skin	LAVENDER + SAGE + ROSEWOOD.
– Hair	LAVENDER + SAGE + THYME + YLANG YLANG. See Sage recipe.
Sinusitis	CHAMOMILE. Lavender, Lemongrass, Eucalyptus.
Sciatica	Lavender + Marjoram + Lemongrass (external).
Shingles	See Rosegeranium recipe.
Skin	
– Care	CARROT, ROSEWOOD, LEMON, ROSE.
– Cleansing	SASSAFRAS, CEDAR. Juniper, Cajuput.
– Revitalising	ROSEMARY, ROSEWOOD, SANDALWOOD, ROSE, Ylang-ylang.
– Anti-wrinkle	ROSEWOOD + ROSE.
– Skin conditions	LEMON, LAVENDER. See Lavender recipe.
Slimming	JUNIPER, BIRCH, ROSEGERANIUM, LEMON.
Smell, loss of	All essential oils diffused in the atmosphere. Basil leaves in infusion.

Illness	Corresponding essential oils
Sores	
– Infected	LAVENDER, CAJUPUT.
– To heal	LAVENDER, ROSEGERANIUM, ROSEMARY. Niaouli, Hyssop.
Spasms	See Anti-spasmodics.
Stiffness	ROSEMARY. Turpentine.
Stiff neck	LAVENDER + MARJORAM + LEMONGRASS. See Pain killers.
Stones	
– Urinary	JUNIPER. Sandalwood, Ylang-ylang, Lemon.
– Bile	JUNIPER, SANDALWOOD, LEMON. Rosemary.
Sprains (ankle)	ROSEMARY. Juniper + clay poultice.
Sunstoke	LAVENDER, ROSEGERANIUM.
Teeth (infection)	CLOVE. See Clove recipe.
Tetanus	See Antiseptics.
Thrush (candida albicans)	OREGANO, THYME, Cinnamon, Savory, Clove.
Toxicity	Mint.
Tuberculosis	CAJUPUT, PINE,THYME, OREGANO.
Ulcers	
– Stomach	LAVENDER + Raw potato juice.
– Varicose	See Circulatory and Antiseptics.
Varicose views	CYPRESS, LEMON.
Vertigo	CHAMOMILE, MINT, LAVENDER.
Vulvitis/vulva-vaginitis	LAVENDER (external).
Warts	THUJA.
Weight loss	See Slimming.
Whitlow	LAVENDER (external). See Antiseptics.
Wounds	LAVENDER.

Plants - Classification

Common name	Primary action	Complementary Action	Essential oil 'type'
BASIL	Tonic	Antispasmodic	...
BERGAMOT	Intestinal infections	Skin conditions	...
CAJUPUT OIL	Chronic lung	Anti-neuralgic infections	...
CHAMOMILE	Antispasmodic	Softener	Sinusitis
CARAWAY	Dyspepsia	Oxygenator	Flatulence
CEDARWOOD	Skin condition	Genito-urinary	...
CINNAMON	Tonic antiseptic	Sexual tonic	Diarrhoea
CITRONELLA	Removes Mosquitoes	...	...
CORIANDER	General tonic	...	...
CLOVE	Anesthetic toothache Tonic for memory	Antiseptic	Toothache Memory
CYPRESS	Circulatory problems	Deep and superficial cellulite. Acne roseace	Circulation
EUCALYPTUS	Sterilises	Fluidifies pulmonary mucus	Respiratory
JUNIPER	Diuretic anti-rheumatism	Slimming	Rheumatism
GINGER	Stimulates glandular functions	Ovaries Testicles	Aphrodisiac
HYSSOP	Chronic pulmonary complaints	Healer – external use	Asthma
LAVENDER	Soothing Skin repair Healer Pulmonary	Regulator of nervous system	Cuts and abrasions. Relaxing.

Common name	Primary action	Complementary Action	Essential oil 'type'
LEMON	General blood purifier	Increases immunities	For women
LEMONGRASS	Tropical antiseptic	...	...
MARJORAM	Anxiety Anguish Insomnia Depression	Soother Regenerator	"Food for nerve cells"
MINT	General and digestive tonic	Refreshing	...
NUTMEG	General and cerebral tonic	Excites the brain and the senses. Digestive	Tonic
NEROLI	Nervous sedative	Cellular revitaliser	Sleep
NIAOULI	Pulmonary antiseptic	...	...
ORANGE	Nervous sedative	Tranquillizer children	Sleep
OREGANO	No. 1 Antiseptic	General tonic	Antibiotic
PETIT GRAIN	Nervous sedative	Tranquillizer	Sleep
PINE	Pulmonary antiseptic	Expectorant	Cough
ROSEMARY	Digestive and tonic	Liver tonic	Tonus for heart sportsmen
ROSE	Anti-cancer	Tissue re-juvenator	No. 1 anti-wrinkle
ROSE GERANIUM	Energises cortical-suprarenal	Healer	Sweet tooth
ROSEWOOD	Tissue regenerator	Toner	Skin
SAGE	Diuretic ovaries regulator	Anti-sweat	Gynaecological

Common name	Primary action	Complementary Action	Essential oil 'type'
SANDAL-WOOD	Genito-urinary antiseptic	Aphrodisiac Skin care	...
SASSAFRAS	Tobacco antidote	...	Anti-tobacco
SAVORY	Genital and intellectual tonic	Improves digestion	Sexual and physical tonic
TARRAGON	Diuretic and ovaries regulator	Anti-sweat	Gynaecological
TURPENTINE	Diuretic	Anti-rheumatism	To perspire
THUJA	Genito-urinary Antiseptic	Warts	Prostatitis
THYME	Powerful Antibiotic		No. 2 antiseptic
VERVAIN	Creates harmony	Increases creativity	Happiness and 'bonheur'
YLANG-YLANG	Sexual tonic	Antiseptic	...

The essential oils listed in column 1 are described as being of a particular 'type' (see column 4) according to my own designation.

For some people, it is enough if they use an essential oil of the correct 'type' for a specific complaint. However, just as there are types of oil which are more effective than others, there are within each type category individual oils which are more effective than others.

For example: Caraway not only *belongs to the type* of oil for treating flatulence, but is also, in all circumstances, the *best* oil for this purpose.

... = no type category.

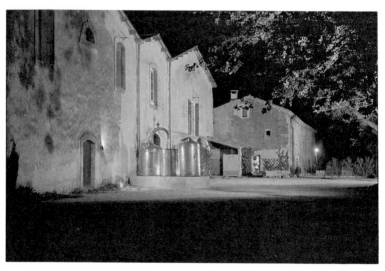

La Chevêche en Provence
Information centre for Holistic Medicine.

CHAPTER 3

Essential Oils for Beauty

The 'Beauty' Pharmacy

Essential oils	Hydrosols	Various
Rosewood	Cornflour	Clay (powder/tube)
Chamomile	Chamomile	Honey
Lemon	Juniper	Seaweeds (powder)
Juniper	Lavender	Chlorumagène
Rose Geranium	Rosemary	Purgative limonette
Lavender	Sage	Castor oil
Rose	Thyme	San pellegrino magnesia
Sandalwood		Wheat germ oil
Sassafras		St John's Wort oil
Sage		Sesame oil
Ylang-ylang		1 mixer
		Some empty bottles
		(brown glass)

Before mixing your preparations relax, loosen up, smile to yourself: it is an enjoyable moment.

Natural aromatic essential oils are delicate but powerful 'friends'. Treat them with consideration, respect and love.

Use the correct quantities.

Always use coloured glass bottles for your preparations and become... the perfect 'pharmacist-alchemist' of your own beauty.

Prepare Your Own Beauty Products
Aromatic Preparations

– Bath oils.
– Body oils/massage oils.
– Frictions of essential oils.
– Face oils/Eyes (outline).
– Hair/feet/nails/oils.
– Vapour treatments/inhalations.
– Masks
– Toilet water/perfumes.
– Aftershave.
– Compresses for eye/burns/vaginal douches/enema.
– Face tonics.

How to Take an Efficient Aromatic Bath

Water temperature:	between 36°C to 40°C, as desired.
Duration:	5 to 30 minutes.
Frequency:	acute illness: 1–2 baths each day.
	chronic illness: 1 bath each day or every other day.
Mandatory rest time:	after each bath: 5–15 minutes.
Aim of bath:	to relax, open up pores and eliminate toxins.

– dip into an aromatic bath at a pleasant temperature.
– relax 5–15 minutes in bath, rub with water.
– when getting out add very hot water for 30 seconds, then get out.
– do not dry yourself, wrap up in a bathrobe.
– lie down with a towel wrapped around your neck, feet and body and cover yourself with a blanket.
– relax for at least 5–15 minutes.
Relaxation and the rush of blood to the surface of the body caused by the last warm phase of the bath, allow for perspiration and the elimination of toxins.
The very short period of high temperature will not affect either the vascular or cardiac systems.
This bathing formula ensures a maximum of efficiency without inconvenience.

If the bath is tonic:
after 5 minutes rest take a cool or cold shower, and rub yourself with a composition of tonic essential oils.

If the bath is relaxing:
continue this relaxation and why not go to sleep relaxed enjoying this well-being all night through?

Bath
All aromatic oils for bathing can be used in showers.
In which case, use natural solvents rather than milky lathers.
Speciality:
When using aromatic body oils of Nelly Grosjean's precious oils (ABO) put 5 drops in bath water.

Aromatic Oils for Baths

Essential oils do not mix with water, they have therefore to be mixed with a natural solvent before introducing them to water, otherwise unpleasant burns will occur!

Only essential oil of Lavender can be used straight in bath water!

– for small children (3–7 years old):	5 drops of essential oil of Lavender in 1 teaspoon of Wheat germ oil.
– for babies: (less than 3 years):	use hydrosol of Lavender – 2 tablespoons per bath.
– for adults:	5–10 drops of essential oil of Lavender or 5–10 drops aromatic oil for bath or 1 glass of hydrosol.

How to Prepare an Oil for Your Bath

In general, 10% to 30% of essential oil is diluted in natural 'solvent'.

Natural 'solvents':	• Wheat germ oil
	• full milk powder
	• seaweed powder
	• egg yolk shampoo
	• neutral foundation

Aromatic oils for baths: in 60ml of Wheat germ oil add:

Cinnamon:	Cinnamon 5ml + Cedar 10ml (optional).
Hindu:	Ylang-ylang 15ml.
Oriental:	Sandalwood 5ml + Rosewood 5ml or Cedar 5ml.
To perspire:	Turpentine 60ml (in 60ml Wheat germ oil).
Tonic:	Rosemary 15ml.
Relaxing:	Marjoram 5ml, Lavender 15ml.
Refreshing:	After sunburn: Lavender 15ml, Mint 5ml or Rosegeranium 10ml + Mint 5ml.
Relaxing:	Rosegeranium 15ml.
Rejuvenating and to combat dry skin:	Rosewood 10ml + Rose Geranium 5ml + Rose 5 drops.
Wood oil to perspire:	Rosewood 5ml + Cedarwood 5ml + Turpentine 30ml + Sandalwood 3ml.
Soothing for children:	Lavender 20ml + Orange 5ml + Mandarin 2ml.
Aphrodisiac:	Lavender 30ml + Ylang-ylang 10ml + Sandalwood 5ml + Rose 5 drops.
Calming:	Chamomile 3ml + Neroli 5 drops + Lavender 20ml.

All essential oils can be used in baths, diluted with a natural 'solvent' 3–10 drops according to oil selected.
For example: Marjoram, Birch, Juniper, Rosegeranium 5–10 drops; Neroli, Vervain, Chamomile 1 drop; Rose ½ drop, Turpentine 10 drops.

Caution: if essential oils are used undiluted in bath water they are liable to 'burn'

Hydrosols for baths   2 tablespoons per bath
Relaxing: Lavender or Chamomile.
Elimination: Juniper.
Tonic: Savory, Rosemary, Oregano.
Fresh: Mint.
Pleasant: Vervain, Marjoram.
Soft: Wild Rose, Lavender, Neroli.

Aromatic Oils for Massage

– aromatic oils (ABOs) for baths and body can be used for massage: they only have to be diluted.
– for different types of massage there are different oils: 'oily', 'greasy' or 'penetrating'.

Dosage 3 – 10% of essential oil for massage

Ingredients

Wheat germ oil:	Rich in vitamin E, rejuvenative, penetrates fast without greasing.
Coconut oil:	Fat, thick, it remains for a while on the surface.
St John's Wort oil:	Double maceration of flowers in olive oil – 0.5% acidity – is said to inflate cartilages (Dr Breuss) and improve blood circulation.
Sesame oil:	Light, fine, penetrates.
Sweet almond oil:	Light, penetrating, becomes rancid fast.

NOTES:

Shiatsu:	*Use essential oil or oils for bath (ABO). Strongly concentrated (30–40% of essential oils in Wheat germ oil.)*
Rolfing-magnetism:	*Apply natural essential oils – see Frictions.*
Californian physiotherapy:	*Use neutral cream, coconut oil, olive oil to which are added Wheat germ oil, St John's Wort oil and essential oils.*

1) Fatty massage oil:	Take 3–5ml essential oil or 10ml aromatic body oils. Add 120ml coconut oil or coconut oil + olive oil in equal parts.
2) Rejuvenative and penetrating massage oil:	Take 3–5ml essential oil or 10ml aromatic oils. Add 60ml Wheat germ oil + 30ml Sesame oil + 30ml St John's Wort oil.

NOTE: Wheat germ oil is rich in vitamin E, excellent for skin, toning and nervous system. Don't forget that any body care product should be 'edible': it is absorbed by the skin and 'digested'.

3) Neutral massage oil:	Take 3–5ml essential oil or 10ml aromatic oils. Add 100ml almond oil or basic neutral cream.

4) Aromatic massage oil for children:
Take 3–10ml essential oil of Lavender, Eucalyptus, Orange or Chamomile or a blend of relaxing aromatic oils. 30ml Wheat germ oil, 30ml Sesame, 30ml Sweet almond oil.

NOTES: Children love Orange and Chamomile! Remember to play with basic oils to obtain the correct fluidity and speed for penetration. Another option: add the selected essential oil to the blend later.

Aromatic Frictions with Essential Oils

Originally, Egyptian perfume was a balm, an ointment, with a flower base prepared by the priest, the physician, the oracle, for the health of body and spirit. My 12 'frictions' restore nature's vital elements, the energy basic to our well being. Use morning or evening to develop physical or mental faculties, love, trust, creativity or communication, much as the 12 moons, 12 months, 12 zodiac signs, 12 apostle... 12 little problems or our daily life. Developed over the past 15 years, they correspond to the 12 metabolic functions of our wonderful body.

A friction with essential oil harmonises, re-balances, tones, relaxes and re-assures: it is our protection just as the fragrance of a flower is its protective envelope.

A friction with essential oil brings a new energy to our body, which is continuously being depleted by life's battles. You will appreciate a friction morning or evening, on the solar plexus, nape of the neck, spine and soles of the feet.

Protection, harmony, vitality, regeneration.

Why use essential oil in frictions?
**– We know that, when essential oils are applied on the skin, within 4
hours the essential oils are in our blood and lymph.**
– Furthermore, the elective property of essential oils gives the following
advantage:
**Essential oils in a friction, or on any part of the body, will inevitably be
attracted to the weak organ or the malfunctioning part.**
We shall therefore talk of 'beauty frictions', those each of us should apply
to increase his/her vital potential and help the body to wake up in the
morning and to relax and sleep well at night.
– tonic morning frictions, evening relaxing, digestive, respiratory,
circulatory, 'pain reliever' or aphrodisiac frictions.
– frictions for the skin, feet, hair.

When to apply frictions

Morning, 6am to 12 noon	Morning tonic.
Evening, 6pm to midnight	Evening relaxing.
5pm and before bedtime	Aphrodisiac.
After the 3 meals	Digestive.
Morning and evening	Respiratory.
Morning, 5pm and before bedtime	Circulatory.
Morning and evening	Feet.

How to apply frictions
– 20 drops in the palm of the hand and apply to the parts to be treated and
to solar plexus.

Where to apply frictions
On the whole body:

Chest, nape of neck, spine, arms, legs, soles of feet and solar plexus:	Tonic, Relaxing, Respiratory.
Tummy, abdomen and solar plexus:	Digestive.
Painful part and solar plexus:	Pain relief.
Feet, legs and solar plexus:	Circulatory.
Feet and legs:	Feet.
Scalp only:	Hair.
Face only:	Face.

How much?

Body frictions:	20–30 drops.
Stomach and abdomen frictions:	15–20 drops.
Pain frictions:	5–10 drops.

Leg frictions:	10–20 drops.
Foot frictions:	10 drops.
Hair frictions:	50–100 drops.
Face frictions:	5–7 drops.
Chest and back frictions:	20–30 drops.

For children with delicate skin:
Frictions must always be mixed with at least an identical volume of Wheat germ, Almond or Olive oil, even if not diluted.
Never use undiluted frictions for infants under 6 months old.

Precautions
The following essential oils can be used as such and not diluted:
Rosewood, Cajuput, Chamomile, Cedar, Lemon, Cypress, Eucalyptus, Juniper, Rosegeranium, Lavender, Marjoram, Myrrh, Niaouli, Orange, Petit grain, Pine, Rosemary, Sandalwood, Ylang-ylang.
Essential oils which must be diluted:
applied directly onto the skin they are liable to burn, chill or simply be unpleasant!
Aniseed, Basil, Bergamot, Cinnamon, Coriander, Tarragon, Ginger, Clove, Lemongrass, Mint, Nutmeg, Neroli, Oregano, Rose, Savory, Sassafras, Sage, Turpentine, Thuja, Thyme, Vervain.

How to dilute them
In essential oil of Lavender, Wheat germ oil or any other basic oil. See Body oils, oils for massages.

Essential Oils: Aromatic Frictions Available from Vie Arome

Properties:

APH action:	Energiser for cortico-adrenal, ideal for fatigue, memory, sexual drive, businessman's stress...
NER relaxation:	Relaxing of the nervous system, favours refreshing sleep, soothes anxieties, worries...
RES breathing:	The ideal winter friction, stops chills, colds, flu, bronchitis, asthma...
RHU pain relief:	Relieves pains, drains kidneys, anti-rheumatism and relieves joints pains...
VIT vitality:	Tonic and vitality. The ideal morning friction, increases punch and dynamism for students, sportsmen and exam time.

106 hair:	Hair regenerative, helps regrowth, tonifies tired limp, brittle, toneless hair.
107 'brilliant feast':	tissue regenerative, strong 'anti-wrinkle' with essential oil of Rose. A genuine 'brilliant feast' for all types of skin.
108 feet:	Circulation, excessive perspiration, heavy legs, hot feet, itching, cellulite, headache, disturbed periods.
CEL cellulite:	Heavy, swollen, tired legs. Difficult circulation, hot and cold feet: in association with 108 friction.
DIG digestion:	Distending, slow and difficult digestion. 'Miracle' cure for flatulence.
MIN slimming:	Elimination, weight control, drains liver and gall bladder.
HAR harmony:	The friction harmoniser of the physical, mental and spiritual. Helps meditation, balance and creativity.

How to use them:
– 20 drops are sufficient as friction, morning and evening, on solar plexus, nape, spine and sole of feet (except 106, 107 an 108 and CEL).
– One 15ml bottle = 6 weeks treatment, morning or evening.

Aromatic Oil for the Face (ABO face)

It's the ideal beauty product, for all, for men and women alike!

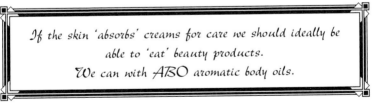

If the skin 'absorbs' creams for care we should ideally be able to 'eat' beauty products.
We can with ABO aromatic body oils.

– Powerful regenerative 'anti-wrinkle' treatment.
ABO face is an aromatic oil specially designed for the face and is the most wonderful products for face care and all types of skin.

Preparation
• 40ml Wheat germ oil
• 20ml St John's Wort oil
• 10ml Sesame oil
• 15ml Rosewood essential oil

• 1 drop essential oil of Rose
apply regularly morning and evening.
NOTES:
– The most regenerative 'anti-wrinkle' treatment, morning and evening
for 3 weeks, then once a day.
– Men enjoy it too!
– 107 friction (see Frictions) 5 – 7 drops patting it in morning and
evening before applying ABO face. Can be used all the year round.
– The ABO face is not greasy: light fine, rich in essential oils,
regenerative in vitamins E, it penetrates immediately.
– For tired blotchy skins:
hydrosol of Sage + friction 107 + ABO face.
– For acne:
hydrosol of Cedar + friction 107 + ABO face or ABO tonic.
Peeling may occur during the first 10 days of use: do not worry, half-
dead cells are eliminated faster and the new skin appears finer,
nourished and regenerated. This is the powerful effect of this 'super'
anti-wrinkle treatment.

Aromatic Oil for the Eye Area
– The best product for the eyes is pure Wheat germ oil.
– One secret: open a capsule of Wheat germ oil and apply by patting it in.
– It's the cheapest and most efficient method on the market!

Aromatic oil for the eye area: toning = ABO eyes.
• Wheat germ oil 90ml
• St John's Wort oil 5ml
• Essential oil of rose 1 drop
• Essential oil of Rosewood 4ml
• Essential oil of Lavender 5ml
NOTES: Should a red spot appear (as often on fragile eye area) dilute
this composition with 100ml Wheat germ oil.

Aromatic Oil for the Hair
To improve dry hair give it an oil bath before shampoo. Leave for 4–12
hours.

Preparation
• 100ml coconut oil
• 30ml Wheat germ oil
• 10ml Ylang-ylang

• 5ml Cedar
• 3ml Thyme
• 5ml Sage.

Shake before use, massage scalp well and coat hair. Olive oil can be used instead of coconut oil.

Note 1: 106* friction is applied to the scalp, and hydrosol of Cedar is added to the aromatic oil for massage, for use as a daily lotion.

Note 2: *For hair loss:*
106* friction + hydrosol of Cedar + Thyme + Sage + live yeast + draining of liver (horseradish and artichoke juice) for 3 – 6 weeks.

Note 3: *Hair rinse after shampoo:*
Hydrosol of Chamomile: for blond hair.
Hydrosol of Cedar: disentangles and softens.
Hydrosol of Cedar + Sage + Thyme + Lavender: for all types of hair.

Note 4: *To eliminate lice:*
Rose Geranium 10ml, Lavender 10ml, Sage 10ml, Thuja 5ml.
20 drops in the evening for 7 days, then once a week for 3 weeks.

Aromatic Oil for the Feet

To relieve 'hot', perspiring red feet.

Preparation:
• 20ml Wheat germ oil
• 80ml Sesame or Olive or Almond oil
• 3ml essential oil of Mint
• 15ml essential oil of Lavender
• 5ml essential oil of Sage.
– Fungi, cold feet, hot feet see 108* friction – feet.
– Hydrosol of Mint refreshes hot feet.

Aromatic Oil for Nails

To revitalise, brittle, broken or soft nails.

Preparation:
– Oil bath 5–10 minutes a day for 1–3 weeks with 1 tablespoon olive oil + lemon juice + 1 drop of essential oil of Lemon.
– Take trace elements, horsetail or nettle juice, both re-mineralisers.

See page 81.

Vapour Treatment

Steam or spray with essential oils to open the pores before treatment.
This is to prepare the skin (face, neck and chest) prior to treatment with a
mask or a regenerative phial.

Preparation:

Vapour treatments are carried out by adding a few drops of essential oils to
steaming hot water.

At home use a bowel of very hot water, inhaler without a nozzle, a
'vapomask' or a container of very hot water to which you will add the
selected essential oils. Put your face above the container and cover your
head with a towel, just as with a steam bath or an inhalation, for 3–4
minutes.

Pre-care, to dilate the pores:

	5–10 drops of essential oil mix.
All skins:	Essential oils of Juniper + Cedar or Sassafras.
Acne:	Essential oils of Juniper + Cedar or Lemon, Sassafras or Thyme + Lemon.

During or after care: to make the pores close:

Dry skins:	Essential oils of Lavender + Rosewood + Rosegeranium.
Acne:	Essential oils of Lavender + Rosewood + Sandalwood.
Wrinkled skins:	Essential oils of Rosemary + Rosewood + Sandalwood.
Flushed skins:	Essential oils of Cypress + Lavender + Rosewood.
Itchy skins:	Essential oils of Rosewood + Lavender + Chamomile.
All skins:	Essential oil of Sage.

Masks

Masks with honey, clay and essential oils cleanse and smooth the face.

Preparation:

1. Honey mask formula:

To 3 tablespoons of honey, add 1–5 drops of essential oils selected for their
desired effect. Mix. Apply to the face, neck and chest with a wooden
spatula.

Keep on for about 7 minutes, rinse with warm water.

2. Mudpack formula:

To 3 tablespoons of fine clay (green, pink or white), add 1–2 drops of
essential oils suitable to your skin. Apply to the face. Keep on for 3–7
minutes while relaxing. As soon as the mask dries, re-apply water or
remove with warm water. Follow with an application of tonic, rejuvenative
phial or cream, according to your needs, or special aromatic oil for the face.

3. Greasy skin formula:
To 2 tablespoonfuls of cold honey, add 2 drops of essential oil of Lemon
and 10 drops of essential oil of Lavender. Apply for 7–10 minutes.
Cleansing mask
3 drops of essential oil of Sassafras, 6 drops Lavender. Add to 2
tablespoons of cold honey.
Mask for all types of skin
2 drops of essential oil of Lemon; mix in powdered clay (green, pink or
white) with enough water to obtain a slightly thick paste. Apply to skin for
7–10 minutes, rinse with water.
Anti-wrinkle mask
Essential oils of Rosemary and Rosewood: 3 drops of each. Add to 2
tablespoons of honey, keep on for 5 minutes. Rinse with warm, then cold
water.

Aftershave

Natural, alcohol-free, rejuvenating and 'anti-wrinkle'.

Aromatic oil tonic	
(ABO tonic):	60ml Wheat germ oil, 30ml St John's Wort oil, 1 drop essential oil of Rose, 20ml Rosemary, 10ml essential oil of Lavender and ½ drop Vervain. Apply a few drops as a non fat oil to nourish skin.
Essential oil of Lavender:	Healing, soothes razor rash: a few drops on the skin.
Lavender hydrosol:	Non-greasy, calms, refreshes.
Aquaderma lotion:	Hydrosols of Lavender, Sage, Thyme, Chamomile, Wild rose, soothe, relax. To be followed with a few drops of ABO tonic or ABO face.

NOTE: Men enjoy the fresh, tonic fragrance of essential oils.

Perfume

Incense – fragrance of the senses...
All perfumes are composed of essential oils – they are the 'foundation' of
all perfumes, called 'base' in France, the land of perfumes.
Ingredients: 70% alcohol, a perfume fixative, some essential oils.
Preparation:
• 15ml of your own essential oil mixture: your 'foundation'.
• 100ml of 70% alcohol.

• 1 tinted glass bottle.

Mix. Add 2 drops clarified Sage: a natural fixative.

Leave to rest for 15 days, away from light and heat.

Filter... then use.

Notes: The same foundation 1–15 ml mixed to 250ml alcohol will produce a toilet water.

– Clarified Sage is a natural vegetable fixative.

– Amber, musk and civet were and still are used in perfumery as fixatives.

– Todays fixatives are often synthetically produced.

Advice and recipes:

In your 'base' use the following sparingly, as they are strongly olfactory:
Cinnamon, Bergamot, Clove, Thyme, Ginger, Oregano, Mint...

To put together your 'base':

– Select soft and flowery oils: Lavender, Vervain, Rosewood, Sandalwood, Lemon, Rose Geranium, Ylang-ylang.

– Add drop by drop (and write them down) the essential oils which inspire you. When using powerful oils you need only $\frac{1}{20}$th of the quantities in the original foundation (Clove, Cinnamon, Neroli, Rose, Ginger...)

– Don't forget to write down your recipe!

Example No. 1: Soft feminine, captivating foundation.

Foundation: Rosegeranium 7ml, Vervain 4ml, Cedar 3ml.

Add: 20 drops of Rose.

Add: 5 drops of Sage as fixative.

Rose Geranium, Vervain and Rose have closely related fragrances which reinforce each other within the same range.

Example No. 2: Heady, oriental, sophisticated foundation.

Foundation: Sandalwood 10ml, Cedar 5ml.

Add: 5 drops of Sage as fixative.

Add: a few drops of Lemon to refresh this oriental foundation or a few drops of Ylang-ylang to make it more Indian.

Face Tonics

Face tonics are prepared from hydrosols, also called hydrolats or floral waters.

Hydrosols are produced from the first 20 litres of water from each distillation of aromatic plants, organically grown and distilled with spring water. Hydrosol is a term devised by Nelly Grosjean to describe this specific quality.

How to use hydrosols

For the face:	Rejuvenating tonic for all skins. Lavender, Thyme, Rosemary, Sage, Wild rose, Carrot, Cedar, Chamomile and Aquaderma...
For razor rash:	Lavender, Rosemary.
For skin conditions and scars:	Cedar + Wild rose + Lavender.
For hair:	Softens, makes silky: Thyme, Cedar. Regrowth: Cedar. After sun: Thyme, Cedar. Blond hair: Chamomile or Chamomile + Thyme.
For baths:	2 tablespoons per bath. Soothing child bath: Lavender, Chamomile. Tonic bath: Thyme, Rosemary. Cheering bath: Vervain.
For eyes:	Softening: cornflour water. Relief: Chamomile.

Some advice on use

Lotions:

Ideal dry skin lotion:	Lavender + Rosemary + Thyme or Wild rose + Chamomile.
Ideal wrinkle lotion:	Rosemary + Sage + Lavender or Aquaderma or Wild rose + Lavender.
Ideal acne lotion:	Cedar or Cedar + Thyme + Lavender.
Ideal lotion for all skins:	Aquaderma.
Ideal lotion for irritated skins:	Lavender + Chamomile.

And more...

As aftershave:	Rosemary + Lavender
As after sun:	Mint + Lavender + Rosemary.
For heavy legs:	Mint.
Hair rinse:	Cedar + Thyme.
Blonde hair:	Chamomile.

NOTE: Don't forget we are speaking about Hydrosols and not about essential oils!

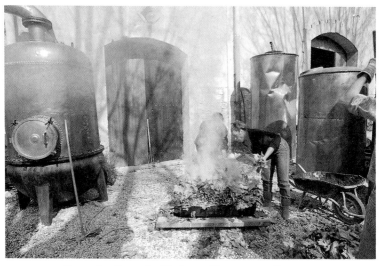

Preparing for a distillation at Graveson en Provence.

CHAPTER 4

Essential Oils in the Kitchen

– Put Together Your Own 'Culinary Pharmacy'
– Summary Table: Essential Oils in the Kitchen
– Recipes
     • cocktails with vegetable juice
     • aromatic oils
     • seasonings
     • vegetable pâtés
– Hydrosols: natural drinks
– Natural 'toddies'

Put Together Your Own 'Culinary Pharmacy'

Essential oils of Lemon, Orange, Mandarin, Tangerine, Cinnamon, Ginger, Bergamot:
for 'healthy' desserts, pureed fruit.
Essential oils of Basil, Tarragon, Coriander:
add to sauces for salads and sprouting beans.
Essential oils of Rosemary, Marjoram, Juniper, Nutmeg, Sage:
for cooked dishes, cereals and vegetable 'pâtés'.
Essential oils of Savory, Cinnamon, Thyme, Rosemary, Coriander, Lemon, Mint, Orange, Marjoram, Pine:
for natural toddies, healthy drinks.

Hydrosol Mint
for sugar-free cordials for children.
Hydrosols Vervain, Sage, Oregano, Savory, Rosemary, Juniper:
for hot or cold healthy drinks.

Notes for Summary Table: Essential Oils in the Kitchen

• Essential oil of Garlic and Onion are never used in cookery: the fresh vegetables themselves are full of fragrance.
• Essence of Rose is rarely used: it's price matches gold!
• Essential oils of Fennel and Dill are not sold to the general public.
• This table shows the suitability of various essential oils or hydrosols for eating or drinking.

For example: as hot or cold drinks: all essential oils and hydrosols can be used; however, as noted, some are more pleasant than others.

Summary Table: Essential Oils in the Kitchen

Essential oil	Essential oil	Hydrosol	Sweets	In salty dishes	Warm drinks	'Health' drinks hydrosols	Fresh drinks syrups	aromatic oils for salad
Basil	•			•				•
Bergamot	•	•	•		•			
Cinnamon	•	•	•		•			
Caraway	•	•		•				
Celery	•					•		
Lemon	•		•		•		•EO	•
Coriander	•		•	•	•			•
Cumin	•			•				
Tarragon	•	•		•		•		•
Fennel	•	•				•		
Juniper	•				•	•		
Rose Geranium	•		•		•			
Ginger	•		•	•	•			
Clove	•		•		•			
Mandarin	•			•		•	•EO	
Marjoram	•	•	•	•	•	•		•
Mint	•	•	•		•	•	•Hyd	•
Nutmeg	•			•	•			
Oregano	•	•		•	•	•	•Hyd	
Orange	•		•	•	•		•EO	
Parsley	•			•		•		
Rosemary	•	•			•	•		•
Sage	•	•		•	•	•	•Hyd	•
Savory	•	•		•	•	•	•Hyd	•
Thyme	•	•		•	•	•		•
Vervain	•	•	•		•	•	•Hyd	

EO = Essential oil
Hyd = Hydrosol

Recipes

Cocktails with vegetable juice

1. EXOTIC COCKTAILS

Andalusian: Tomato, cucumber, pepper + 1 drop essential oil of Mint.

Caribbean: Carrot, pepper + lime juice (fresh).

Mexican: Carrot, tomato, pepper + lime juice (fresh) + pimento water + 1 drop essential oil of Ginger.

Indian: Carrot, green cabbage + 1 drop essential oil of Cinnamon.

African: Carrot, cabbage, courgette + 1 drop essential oil of Coriander + 1 drop essential oil of Caraway.

Provence: Carrot, tomato + 1 drop essential oil of Basil.

Hawaiian: (Very strong) Carrot, courgette, pepper + 1 tablespoon of decoction (Ginger) + 1 teaspoon pimento water.

2. COCKTAILS FROM THE FRENCH PROVINCES

Midi: Carrot, Celery + 1 drop essential oil of Basil or Coriander.

Basque: Carrot, Tomato, Cucumber + 1 drop of essential oil of Nutmeg.

Alsace: Carrot, Green cabbage + 1 drop essential oil of Caraway.

Riviera: Carrot, Celery, Cucumber + 1 drop essential oil of Tarragon.

3. CLEANSING COCKTAILS

Excellent for the liver: ¼ carrot, ¼ radish + 1 drop essential oil of Rosemary.

Excellent for the kidneys: ½ carrot, ½ celery + 1 drop essential oil of Juniper.

Excellent for the stomach: ⅓ carrot, ⅓ green cabbage, ⅓ potato + 1 drop essential oil of Tarragon.

4. TO HELP WITH NURSING MOTHERS AND FOR CLEANSING KIDNEYS: Fennel.

5. TO REDUCE GENERAL ACIDITY AND LOSE WEIGHT:

Watermelon or carrot + watermelon or fennel or carrot + radish.

Summing up: For 1 litre of vegetable juice: 3–4 drops essential oil.

– The carrot or tomato base makes half, the other vegetables make up the other half of the mixture.

– Only radish is to be added with 5–10 small radishes or 5cm horseradish to 1 litre of carrot juice.

– Onion: ¼ onion in a litre of carrot juice.

– Strongly flavoured vegetables are added in small quantities: celery,

radish, leek, onion, potato: 1 tablespoon per glass of juice.
– to add essential oils (3–7 drops per litre of juice): place the oil on top of the vegetables in a liquidiser.
– Seasoning (herbal, ginger, saffron or pimiento water) is added when serving.
– A vegetable juice can be kept for 4–5 hours in a refrigerator. Stir before serving.
– There is no limit to drinking vegetable juice (1 or 2 litres per day without any problem, during a course of treatment).
Remember: fresh vegetable juices 'densify', re-mineralise, tone and nourish.
– Vegetable juices are real food.
– You can follow a simple diet of vegetable juices for a few weeks.
– Treatment with vegetable juices is ideal in cases of serious illness.
– The tea-break 'aperitif of vegetable juice' is sacred just as with traditional drinks. The result is: calm, relaxation, smiling faces.
• *The one food diet: take one single daily food, several times a day. This can be just vegetable juice (1–3 litres). It is wonderfully cleansing, whilst making you feel full of vital energy.*

Aromatic Oils with Essential Oils

How to prepare them:
Prepare ¼ of first cold-pressed olive oil to which are added: 6 drops essential oils of Basil or Coriander or Tarragon or Caraway or Cumin (3 drops only) + fresh pimiento and sea salt (optional) or herbamare.
To be used as a salad dressing.
Essential oils of Basil, Caraway, Cumin, Coriander, Juniper, Rosemary, Mountain savory, Bay leaf, Tarragon, Nutmeg, Marjoram, Oregano can be added: 1 drop in the dressing for each handful of sprouting beans per person and for 4 people.
Note: The olive oil can be replaced in full or in part with yoghurt, cream cheese or avocado.

Seasonings
Sea salt with oil, tamarisk, yeast, vegetable extract (powdered), pimiento, cider vinegar, lemon, lime, paprika go together in dressings for sprouting beans.
Other seasonings worth mentioning:
Sunflower seeds soaked (15 minutes), ground hazelnuts or almonds, olive 'purée'... give much variety to seasonings.

Vegetable pâtés

A good way not to waste beans that have been sprouting for 2–3 days: Put them in the mixer with some vegetable juice (carrot, fennel, courgette...), add olive oil and yeast. Season with fresh herbs, basil, tarragon, parsley, garlic onion... and/or some essential oils and serve immediately.

Recipes and essential oil allowance for 6 persons
– whilst cooking:

Cumin, Caraway, Coriander, Nutmeg, Thyme, Marjoram, Sage, Rosemary to be added to a maximum of 4/8 drops.

Example:

– To pasta 1: add 1 drop Juniper, 1 drop Caraway, 3 drops Basil.
– To pasta 2: add 3 drops Tarragon, 1 drop Juniper.
– To pasta 3: add 2 drops Coriander, 1 drop Juniper.
– To pickles: add 4 drops Juniper, 1 drop Caraway, 1 drop Coriander.
– To stews (vegetable or meat): Thyme, Bay leaf, Coriander, Laurel, Nutmeg, Sage and Rosemary adding up to less than 8 drops altogether.

When serving:

Adjust your seasoning of salt, pepper, pimiento, curry, saffron according to the dish, using 1–2 drops maximum of the selected essential oils. They will give the finishing touch to your dish.

Adding the essential oils at the last moment will bring out the fullness of their aroma as they will not be over-heated.

Hydrosols

Some advice on their use

Quality
Vie Arôme's hydrosols are produced from the first 20 litres of water of each distillation of aromatic plants. The plants are organically grown and are distilled with spring water. 'Hydrosol' is a specific name used by Nelly Grosjean for a specific 'natural floral water' or 'hydrolat'.

How to use them

On the face, as a lotion:
– Rejuvenator, tonic for all skins: Lavender, Thyme, Rosemary, Sage, Carrot, Cedar, Chamomile and Aquaderma.
Razor rash: Lavender, Rosemary.
Skin conditions and scars: Cedar.
Hair, as a hair lotion, every day:
– Soften: Thyme, Cedar.
– Growth: Cedar.
– After sun: Thyme, Cedar.
– Blond hair: Chamomile.
Bath: 2 tablespoons per bath:
Soothing bath for children: Lavender, Chamomile.
Tonic bath: Thyme, Rosemary, Oregano, Savory.
These are hydrosols, not essential oils which are liable to 'burn'.
Eyes, as lotion:
– Soothing: cornflour water.
– Relief: Chamomile.
Drink:
Hydrosols are the new 'liquid' herbal teas and the 'daily health treatment drink': Sage, Mint, Oregano, Thyme, Eucalyptus, Juniper...
2 tablespoons in 1½ litre. Drink the mixture each day or 1 teaspoon in a cup of warm water.
Cooking:
Add to vegetable juice, soups, seasonings, salad dressings, sorbets...

'Hydrosols' are a speciality of Vie Arôme. To order, write to;
Aromathérapie Vie Arôme
La chevêche – petite route du grès
13690 – Graveson en Provence
France
Telephone: 90 95 81 72 – Fax: 90 95 85 20

Natural 'Toddies' with Essential Oils

Type A:

Anti-flu and tonic:
Oregano, Thyme, Cinnamon, Clove, Rose Geranium, Ginger (optional), 1 drop of each on a large spoon of honey, juice of lemon and a large cup of hot water. Can be taken 2–3 times a day without trouble.

Anti-cough:
Pine, Eucalyptus, Orange, 1 drop of each on a spoonful of honey, hot water and lemon juice. If necessary, drink 2–3 times a day.

Memory cocktail:
Clove, Coriander, Rosemary, 1 drop of each, in a large glass of water and 1 spoonful of mint honey.

Asthma cocktail:
Thyme, Hyssop, Chamomile, Cajuput. A drop of each on a spoonful of honey, warm water. Serve with ice cubes.

Anti-tobacco cocktail:
Sassafras, Sage, Rose Geranium, Marjoram, Lavender, 1 drop of each in a spoonful of honey and a large glass of water water served with ice cubes and a dash of mint cordial.

Aphrodisiac cocktail:
Savory, Ceylon cinnamon, Clove, Rosemary, Rose Geranium, 1 drop of each on a spoonful of honey in a glass of warm water, to be served with ice cubes as a long drink. A dash of mint syrup or mint hydrosol can be added to this cocktail.

Type B:

Special good digestion drinks:
Clove, Ginger or Coriander, Oregano, 1 drop of each on a spoonful of honey and in a large glass of warm water, every 2 hours. You could also use 3 drops of Mint.

Type C:

Refreshing drinks:
Cedar, Rose Geranium or Lemon: 1 drop of each on a spoonful of honey in a large glass of warm or cold water or 3 drops of mint essential oil.

Life is joy.
Giono

*Joy is proof that what
you live is good.*
Hindu saying

*Joy is all, it's up to us
to discover it.*
Confucius

LA CHEVECHE
Graveson en Provence – France

A place to visit and collect information on aromatherapy, perfumes and natural medicines, between the Alpilles and the Montagnette, close to les Baux de Provence, in the heart of the countryside.

1) Organic cultivation of aromatic plants.

2) Distillation of essential oils and hydrosols.

3) Vie Arôme's aromatherapeutic laboratory: production and distribution, mail order, worldwide.

4) Health school and lectures open to the public.

5) Advice, consultation, lectures and training in aromatherapy and holistic medicine, naturopathy and rolfing.

6) Musée de arômes et du parfum: conducted tours for groups or individuals.

7) Aromatherapy and perfume boutique.

8) Publishing of note books and books: holistic medicine and aromatherapy.

9) Health food restaurant in the main house 'mas', lunch, tea and healthy natural drinks.

Nelly Grosjean – La Chevêche. Telephone 90 95 81 55 Fax: 90 95 85 20.

In the U.S.A.
Vie Arôme's products are distributed by;
Aromatherapy International,
Three Seal Harbor Road, Suite 437,
Winthrop, MA 02152
tel: 617 846 0285   fax: 617 846 5474

Visit the 'Musée des Arômes et du Parfum' Graveson en Provence

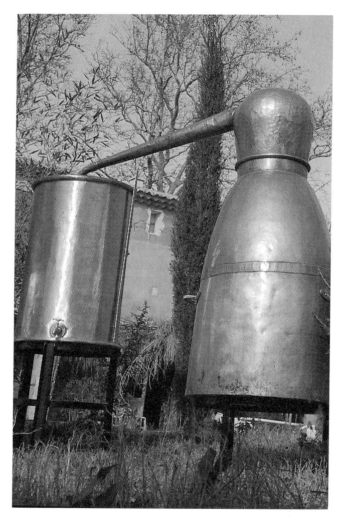

Early 19th century lavender copper still known as 'Tête de Mores' (Moor's head), musée des arômes et du parfum, 13690 – Graveson en Provence, France.

La Chevêche
Petite Route du Grès, 13690 Graveson en Provence, France
Telephone: 033 90 95 81 55. Fax: 033 90 95 85 20.

Index

Index

The ideal beauty product for everyone!
If the skin "absorbs" creams, then you should be able to "eat" beauty
products – that's what happens when you use aromatic body oils!

Aromatic Body Oils
Nelly Grosjean's precious oils

Aromatic body oils can be used:
– in the bath (5 to 6 drops are sufficient)
– in oil applied to the body (prevents dryness of the skin)
– on the face and around the eyes.

Aromatic body oils are gentle and delicate on all skin types, and contain
pure essential oil of rose, known for its regenerative properties.
Aromatic body oils consist of oils from cereal grains, fruit or herbs in
synergy with essential aromatic oils (30 to 40%).
Entirely natural products without preservatives or chemicals of any kind.
Rich in noble vitamins, their active aromatic properties make these oils
remarkable for their regenerative, anti-aging and revitalising qualities.
True aromatic beauty oils, they can be diluted in a neutral massage oil base
for regular use.
St John's wort softens the texture of the skin.
Wheatgerm oil contains vitamin C and tones the skin. The remarkable
essence of rose imparts to these beauty oils an extraordinary regenerative
and anti-aging action.

ABO tonic: for use in the morning, tones and stimulates (with
               rosemary)
ABO relax: for the evening, relaxes
ABO fresh: after exposure to the sun, for legs that feel "heavy",
               refreshing (with mint)
ABO comfort: as a beauty oil, soothing (with geranium)
ABO face: especially for the face, "anti-wrinkle", tones and firms
ABO eyes: specially for around the eyes, soft and soothing

Nelly Grosjean's aromatic body oils are manufactured by the Vie 'Arôme
laboratory, and the quality is therefore guaranteed.

Natural essential oil massage preparations

Perfumed oil was originally used in Egypt as a balm or ointment made from flowers or plants prepared by the priest, doctor or oracle, for the health of the body and spirit. It can be used in the morning or evening to promote physical and mental wellbeing, loving qualities, confidence, creativity or communication. Just as there are 12 moons, 12 months, 12 signs of the zodiac and 12 apostles, so there are the 12 minor problems of daily life. My 12 massage preparations, developed over more than 15 years, correspond to the 12 metabolic functions of our remarkable human body.

An essential oil massage preparation harmonises, balances, tones, relaxes and soothes; as the perfume envelops the flower, so these oils protect us from the rigours of daily life and bring our body vital, renewed energy.

With their properties of protection, harmony, vitality and regeneration, my 12 massage preparations both store and restore nature's vital elements, bringing us extra energy essential for our well-being. You will enjoy the benefits of them both morning and evening.

My 12 massage preparations...in synergy with natural essential oils

APH action: *Cinnamon, coriander, cloves, nutmeg, pine, rosemary, savory, thyme, ylang-ylang*
Mental alertness, physical equilibrium, memory, sexual drive, cellular vitality

NER relax: *Rosewood, lavender, lemongrass, marjoram, bitter orange*
Inner peace, promotes sleep

HAR harmony: *Rosewood, camomile, sandalwood, rose*
Relaxation, meditation, yoga

RES respiration: *Eucalyptus, cajeput oil tree, lavender, pine, rosemary*
Purification of respiratory tract, stimulation of natural immune system

RHU pain relief: *Birch, juniper, marjoram, pine, rosemary*
Relief of pain

CEL cellulite: *Rosewood, birch, cypress, lavender, rosemary*
Toning up veins, disinfiltration of soft tissue

VIT vitality: *Coriander, rose geranium, lavender, pine, nutmeg, rosemary*
Success in exams and competitions, increased drive and dynamism

DIG digestion: *Caraway, coriander, cumin, nutmeg*
Good digestion

MIN slimming: *Lemon, juniper, rose geranium, sandalwood*
Detoxification of the body, weight control

106 hair: *Cedar, lavender, sage, thyme, ylang-ylang*
Promotes beautiful hair, stimulates hair follicle, prevents greasy hair

107 masterpiece: *Rosewood, lavender, rose, sandalwood*
Powerful tissue regenerator, No.1 "anti-wrinkle" remedy

108 legs/feet: *Rosewood, cypress, lavender, mint, sage*
Warms up cold feet, promotes good peripheral circulation, refreshes, relieves legs that feel "heavy"

20 drops will be sufficient – rub in morning and evening on the solar plexus, nape of the neck, spine, and soles of the feet (except 106, 107, 108, CEL).
One 15ml bottle will be sufficient for 6 weeks of treatment, morning or evening.

Quality

Vie 'Arôme hydrosols are produced from the first 20 litres of water from each distillation of aromatic plants, untreated and distilled at source. All Vie 'Arôme hydrosols are made from plants grown organically at Sault. A slight sediment may occur after a few months, in which case filtering will be all that is required.

Vie'Arôme hydrosols

How do I use them?

- as a daily drink: *sage, mint, oregano, savory, thyme, eucalyptus, juniper*
  2 tablespoons in 1½ litres of water per day
- as a rapid infusion: *mint, sage, rosemary, oregano, savory, thyme, verbena*
  1 teaspoon per cup of hot (not boiling) water
- as a "sugarfree" syrup: *mint, verbena*
  2 to 4 tablespoons per litre of water (+ fructose or honey if required)
- for the bath (2 tablespoons per bath):
  - calms children being bathed: *lavender, camomile,*
  - as a bath tonic: *thyme, rosemary, oregano, savory*
- for the hair (as a lotion):
  - makes soft and silky: *thyme, cedar*
  - aids regrowth: *cedar*
  - after sun: *thyme, cedar*
  - for blond hair: *camomile or camomile and thyme*
- for the eyes (as a compress):
  - soothes: *corn-flower water*
  - as a decongestant: *camomile*
- for smarting skin after shaving: *lavender, rosemary*
- for the face:
  - regenerative, tonic for all skin types: *lavender, thyme, rosemary, sage, eglantine, cedar, camomile and aquaderma*

The aromatic diffuser

Regenerates, purifies, perfumes, ionises and enriches the air you breathe. Electrically powered, the aromatic diffuser disperses into the air thousands of micro particles of essential oil, without heating them and through an ingenious system of cold air vaporisation, consisting of a pump and a clear pyrex container. You can use this diffuser to change the olfactory decor of your home whenever you wish.

Essential oils used in the diffuser

- to calm and soothe   lavenders, orange, aids relaxation harmony, bio relax environment
- to tone and stimulate   tonic freshtonic bio fresh environment
- to aid breathing   respiratory, bio respir tonic environment, Christmas environment
- the environments   anti-tobacco environment, Christmas exotic verbena environment

Exotic verbena is our "essential oil for happiness", ideal for promoting communication and to be enjoyed by everyone!

Further information on request from
Vie 'Arôme, La Chevêche, 13690
Graveson en Provence, France.
Tel: 033 90 95 81 72. Fax: 033 90 95 85 20.